10 Ways to Live Longer

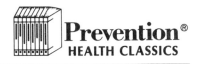
Prevention® HEALTH CLASSICS

10 Ways to Live Longer

by the Editors of Prevention® Magazine

Written and compiled by

Sharon Faelten

With contributions by

Stefan Bechtel
Dominick Bosco
Mark Bricklin
Donna L. Danielson
Mark Diamond
John Feltman
William Gottlieb
Emrika Padus
Kerry Pechter

Linda Shaw
Carl Sherman
Porter Shimer
Tom Stoneback
Jonathan Uhlaner
Tom Voss
Julian M. Whitaker, M.D.
John Yates

Martha Capwell, Research Associate

Rodale Press, Emmaus, Pennsylvania

NOTICE

If you are taking prescription drugs or suffer from a serious ailment, we advise you to seek medical consultation before making any major changes in your diet or beginning an exercise program.

Library of Congress Cataloging in Publication Data

Faelten, Sharon.
   10 ways to live longer.
   (Prevention health classics)
   Includes index.
   1. Health. 2. Longevity. I. Prevention
(Emmaus, Pa.) II. Title. III. Title: Ten
ways to live longer. IV. Series.
RA776.5.F26   613   81-19905
ISBN 0-87857-380-1 paperback   AACR2

   4   6   8   10   9   7   5   3   paperback

Contents

Introduction

Scientists now estimate that nature designed our bodies to last about 120 years. Yet the life expectancy for most people is about 74 years. That means most of us will live out less than two-thirds of our potential life span.

What is it that chops off one-third of our lives? A few decades ago, when people lived even shorter lives, it was infectious diseases, such as tuberculosis. But medical science and improved living conditions have checked the most common deadly bugs. Now it's *degenerative* diseases—heart disease, cancer and stroke—that account for about 75 percent of the deaths in this country. (Accidents, bronchitis and respiratory problems, pneumonia and influenza, diabetes, cirrhosis of the liver, atherosclerosis and suicide make up most of the other 25 percent.) In many ways, however, the change from infectious to degenerative diseases is fortunate. Because the more scientists learn about degenerative diseases, the more they discover that we actually have a great deal of control over their occurrence. In fact, the Surgeon General announced in 1979 that at least seven of the ten leading causes of death in the United States could be substantially reduced through commonsense changes in the lifestyle of many Americans.

What kinds of changes? For starters, weight control, regular meals and regular exercise, enough sleep each night, no smoking, moderate or no drinking and moderate snacking. A study conducted in Alameda County, California, showed that men who followed at least six of these seven health practices lived an average of 11 years longer than men who practiced fewer than four. And women who followed at least six of the health habits lived an average of 7 years longer than women who followed fewer than four *(Preventive Medicine, March, 1973.)*

Keys to Slower Aging

That study is even more encouraging when you find out
vi that many of those commonsense steps—and others discussed

throughout this book—not only lengthen life, but keep you spry and alert in your later years. In fact, if you follow them you may find out that "normal" aging is abnormal.

Ask a gerontologist—a specialist in the aging process—what normally happens when a person grows older, and he'll tell you a horror story. Muscle is replaced by fat. Bones grow thin and fragile. Strength ebbs. Nerve signals slow down. Arteries stiffen and clog with plaque. Defense against infection weakens. And the brain shrinks, losing at least one-tenth of its weight.

Well, all that happens to *some* people. But not to everyone. There are folks who work a 40-hour week and exercise regularly—and enjoy life—into their eighties and beyond. They're not decrepit by any stretch of the imagination. They've learned—through experience—that aging is more a decision than a decree.

For instance, must the brain shrink with age? According to a professor at the University of California at Berkeley, the answer is probably not. Marion Diamond, Ph.D., found that old rats *increased* their brain sizes when given stimulating environments—a larger than average cage, other rats to pal around with and challenging gizmos to manipulate. And while old rats aren't old people, the professor believes her finding—that enjoyment restores the brain—probably holds true for us humans, too.

And the evidence is on her side. Studies of people show that folks who are deeply involved with others, greatly enjoy their work or develop their creativity live longer than people who are detached, dissatisfied or unproductive.

But control over health and longevity doesn't stop with the brain. Throughout this book you'll read how *every* part of the body can be kept young if you have healthy habits. Bones and muscles thrive on exercise, even in later years. You can bolster your immunity by taking vitamins and minerals. Arteries stay clearer on a low-fat diet. Memories stay sharper if you don't smoke. And learning to cope with stress can add years to your life.

So the message is, it's not time alone that ages a body. How fast we age—and how soon we die—is the result of whether we have more health pluses than health minuses. Among the pluses are a nutritious diet, plenty of activity, and a positive attitude. Some of the minuses are a diet high in fat, salt and sugar; smoking and too much drinking; and letting stress get the best of us. When we let the pluses outnumber the minuses, we can live not only longer but fuller and more active lives. To learn more about the ten pluses that will boost your chances of living—and living it up—well beyond the 74-year average, read on.

PART I

Shaping Up for Longevity

Lose Weight— and Gain Years

CHAPTER 1

At the height of World War I, Denmark's foreign trade was cut off by patrolling warships. Food shortages forced most Danes to subsist on a very simple diet. Pork and beef were so scarce and expensive that few Danes ate more than four ounces of meat a day. They lived mostly on bran bread, barley soup, potatoes, greens and milk. In short, Danes ate less than before and lost weight. And, as later studies showed, they lived longer.

Reporting in a postwar volume of the *Journal of the American Medical Association* (February 7, 1920), Dr. M. Hundhede of the Laboratory for Nutrition Research in Copenhagen noted that, before food rationing, the Danish death rate had remained unchanged since 1900. But during the years of food scarcity (1917 and 1918) the death rate among men dropped significantly—34 percent in Copenhagen and approximately 17 percent in all of Denmark.

During World War II, the same thing happened. German occupation of Scandinavia sharply limited butter, milk, cheese and egg consumption. As a result, dietary fats were reduced by half—and the number of deaths from arteriosclerosis (hardening of the arteries) and heart disease dropped by more than 35 percent. A return to the traditional high-fat diet after the war promptly raised death rates to prewar levels.

But food habits—and civilian longevity—can be improved without war. Five Belgian universities have urged Belgians to declare the dietary equivalent of war. The mass media joined the campaign in 1970. As a result, Belgians have voluntarily cut down on fat and cholesterol. A study of 10,000 families, begun in 1967, revealed that the new Belgian diet—like the Scandinavian low-fat diet of World War II—decreased the incidence of heart disease. And like the Danes of World War I, the Belgians were living longer—an average of more than two years longer (*Lancet*, May 21, 1977).

Declare War on Your Diet

In direct contrast to Europeans on wartime diets, Americans tend to overeat—and live far shorter lives. The average American, for instance, eats 10 percent more food than he or she did during World War II, and over 20 percent more than during World War I. And it shows: overweight is a major health problem. There's no question, too, that those extra pounds are life-shortening.

The Alameda County study (mentioned in the Introduction) showed that people who were more than 20 percent overweight died at a younger age than those who were not overweight.

Another study showed that among 200 extremely overweight men, degenerative diseases such as heart disease showed up at an earlier age, progressed more rapidly and became life-threatening more often than in people of normal weight. Heavy people also tended to suffer more fatal accidents such as auto crashes, drowning and choking. (*Journal of the American Medical Association*, February 1, 1980).

Diana Woodruff, Ph.D., associate professor of psychology at Temple University, Philadelphia, measured 32 factors known to be associated with longevity. She, too, found overweight to be a major obstacle to long life. "People who live to be 100 tend to be able to push themselves away from a meal before they are full," said Dr. Woodruff.

What all those scientific studies and observations add up to is this: eating wisely to stay slim is a top priority in achieving longer life. And it's never too late to start. If you're overweight now, chances are that losing extra pounds will:

- take strain off your heart and lower blood fats, reducing the risk of fatal heart attack;
- lower your blood pressure, decreasing your chances of suffering a fatal stroke;
- lower your chances of developing breast cancer, if you're a woman;
- help normalize your blood sugar, which cuts down the risk of developing maturity-onset (adult-onset) diabetes—and makes the condition far less life-threatening if you already have it;
- decrease your chances of having a serious accident.

Best yet, perhaps, slenderizing will make you feel better, look younger, and give you new confidence and optimism—all decisive factors in a longer life.

Choosing the Right Foods Helps Weight Loss

The main thing is to cut down on two common high-calorie substances: sugar and fat. A first step toward that goal is to eat fewer processed foods, for if they're not overloaded with fat, they're probably drenched with sugar (and may have plenty of both). A second step is to choose less fatty versions of common foods—poultry and fish instead of beef, for instance, or skim milk instead of whole. A third step is to increase your intake of natural, whole foods, such as fruits, vegetables and grains, all of which are low in fat. And the best whole foods—at least as far as your waistline is concerned—are those that are packed with complex carbohydrates.

Wait a minute! Aren't carbohydrates—potatoes, beans, rice, corn and the lot—fattening? No, that's a myth that needs debunking. A boiled potato, for instance, has the same number of calories as an apple. It's *refined* carbohydrates in foods like corn chips and doughnuts that are fattening because you can stuff yourself with them without feeling full. But complex carbohydrates are high in fiber, the "roughage" that keeps your bowels working smoothly. And fiber not only fills you up, it actually reduces the amount of calories you absorb from food.

A study by the U.S. Department of Agriculture (USDA) and the University of Maryland revealed that when we eat a diet moderately high in fiber, we absorb about 5 percent fewer calories than when we eat a typical low-fiber diet. That 5 percent reduction will mean, on the average, about 100 fewer calories absorbed and converted into fat each day. And that 100-calorie reduction is accomplished without any whole grains in the diet. There's good reason to believe that if we follow a truly high-fiber diet—one that includes plenty of bran (the fiber from whole wheat), whole grains, beans and peas—the number of calories we can save each day could easily reach 150. And *that* could mean losing ten pounds a year without even trying! (For more details on other life-extending properties of fiber, see the chapter Put Fiber to Work for You.)

Take Your Time

The worst possible way to slim down is to lose weight rapidly. Constant calorie counting, deprivation and willpower battles may help shave off pounds quickly, but sooner or later we're back to our old eating habits, and as fat as ever. The only realistic way of staying slender is to build new habits that will automatically help keep us at our desired weights. Pounds that drop off slowly *stay* off. What's more, we feel better; no starvation, no light-headed feeling, no jumpy nerves.

Here's how to adopt a diet you can truly live with:

FIRST TWO WEEKS. Select one item you know you are over-indulging in and resolve not to eat it more than once a week. Choose something like ice cream, pie, cookies, beer or soda. And instead munch on something like a carrot or a couple of plain crackers. Or drink some herb tea or carbonated water with lemon. That's all you do to your diet for the first two weeks.

Also get some exercise. The easiest way to do that is to begin taking short daily walks. Begin with 15 minutes, and increase your walking time gradually. (For more on exercise, see the next chapter, Exercise Now.)

SECOND TWO WEEKS. Select one more high-calorie item and don't eat it more than once a week. Carry on with the habits of the first two weeks.

SECOND MONTH. Every two weeks drop another snack, so at the end of this month, you'll have eliminated four fat foods, but still enjoy the luxury of "indulging" once a week. Eat anything else you please.

THIRD MONTH. Gradually cut down on butter, mayonnaise and deep-fried foods, so that by the end of this month you're eating only half your usual amount of those items. Carry on with all your earlier habit changes.

FOURTH MONTH. Cut out second helpings, except on Sunday. That's the only change you make this month. And don't forget your daily stroll or other workout.

FIFTH MONTH. Apply the "only-once-a-week" rule to two more snack items. By the end of the month you'll have controlled your eating of a total of six fattening items that aren't so good for your health anyway.

By this time, the battle has been largely won — but without any real struggle with your appetite. Your new habits will have taken firm hold as your excess weight has been slipping away. Carry on with those habits in the weeks ahead, and your weight will probably stabilize anywhere from about 20 to 40 pounds under what it was when you began. And it'll stay there, too, with no big effort.

Exercise Now

CHAPTER 2

Any mechanic will tell you that keeping your car tuned up will lengthen its life expectancy. Well, the same goes for your body. And exercise, as it turns out, tunes us up for a longer, *better* life.

In addition to improving our muscle tone and self-image, honest-to-goodness vigorous exercise has been shown to:

- improve weight control,
- strengthen bones,
- lower blood pressure,
- lower triglycerides (blood fats that doctors believe are bad),
- increase the level of high-density lipoproteins—HDL (the good type of cholesterol),
- improve heart output and efficiency,
- improve the oxygen-carrying capacity of the blood,
- lower blood sugar,
- regulate insulin release,

and *all* of those are conducive to a long and active life.

On the other side of the ledger, *inactivity* lowers your odds for long life. Ralph S. Paffenbarger Jr., M.D., from the California Department of Health, said that lack of exercise *doubles* the risk of premature death from heart disease for people with, for instance, high blood pressure, a previous heart attack or a cigarette habit. Clearly, the risks of inactivity are too threatening to take sitting down.

Your Whole Body Stays Younger with Exercise

You're only as old as your individual parts. Exercise keeps our most vital tissues at their very best in spite of age.

MUSCLES STAY YOUNG. Muscles don't have to age. "You can increase or maintain muscle mass as you get older," said Lawrence E. Lamb, M.D., a cardiologist and noted medical columnist. As a matter of fact, muscle mass will decline with age *only if the body isn't exercised.*

BONES DON'T BREAK. Muscles aren't the only tissues that thrive on exercise. Bones also need movement to stay thick and strong. That's why exercise could help millions of people avoid osteoporosis, a disease in which bones lose their density and become weak. But osteoporosis does more than slow you down—it can stop you cold. As many as six million people in the United States have it, most of them women over 60, and an estimated 100,000 of those women break their hips every year. Almost half of these *don't live more than a year beyond their falls,* according to Everett L. Smith, Ph.D., assistant clinical professor at the University of Wisconsin Center for Health Sciences, in Madison. So having strong bones not only keeps you young—it may keep you alive.

But osteoporosis doesn't happen overnight. "Between the ages of 30 and 70, women lose 30 percent of their bone structure," said Dr. Smith. "Men, on the other hand, don't begin to lose bone until age 55 and don't have significant bone loss until their eighties."

Yet bone loss isn't inevitable, said Dr. Smith. He believes *inactivity* is a big part of the problem, and *activity* a big part of the solution.

Dr. Smith said that exercise is a major factor in keeping the minerals necessary for strength *in* bones, rather than letting age drain them away. As a matter of fact, physical activity can actually increase bone mineral content and strengthen bones beyond normal, according to Dr. Smith. He explained that bones respond to exercise in the same way that muscles do—they become bigger and stronger when more stress is placed on them.

"Bone adapts like any other body tissue," he told us. "When stressed it builds up and becomes stronger; when not stressed it becomes smaller and wastes away. Two forces—gravitational force and muscular activity—act on bone to stress it. These two forces in combination cause bone to become stronger. You force your bones to adapt."

Research bears out that concept. "Current research on tennis players demonstrates that a right-handed tennis player's right arm contains 30 percent more bone than the left arm, which doesn't get used as much," Dr. Smith told us. "Other research shows a person's bone mass can also depend on which type of sport he or she plays. Weight lifters show more bone buildup than throwers, throwers more than runners, and runners more than swimmers."

Applying that to the problem of osteoporosis, Dr. Smith conducted a three-year study of 80 women over the age of 80 in whom exercise slowed the degenerative process of that disease. He then set up an experiment with three groups of women: one that took calcium supplements, one that exercised as a group and one that continued life as usual. The calcium group took 750 milligrams of calcium every day. (That equals the calcium found in about 2½ cups of milk.) The physical-activity group exercised 30 minutes per day, three times a week. After three years the control group—who didn't change their lifestyle—had lost bone, while both the calcium group and the exercise group actually *gained* a small amount of bone mass. And the exercise group gained the *most* bone—about 5.5 percent more than the control group.

"I think this shows the dire need to participate in physical activity a minimum of three days per week for 30- to 40-minute periods," Dr. Smith concluded. He thinks that some bone loss comes with age regardless of what you do, but *you can reduce the loss between the ages of 30 and 70 by as much as half with proper diet and exercise.*

(For more on calcium and bone strength, see the chapter Supplements for the Best Years of Your Life.)

SKIN STAYS FIT. People who exercise regularly may have thicker, stronger skin, according to a Finnish study. That means exercise may slow down the aging of the skin. Researchers compared 50 runners and cross-country skiers who trained about 30 miles a week to 50 healthy but untrained men. They found that the trained men's skin was thicker and more flexible (*British Journal of Dermatology*, August, 1978). But does exercise actually prevent skin from aging? For those who exercise, a look in the mirror may be all the evidence required.

YOUR HEART LOVES TO EXERCISE. Despite what many people believe, heart disease is not "normal" in old people. "Aging itself does not appear to cause cardiovascular disease," said Jeffrey S. Borer, M.D., formerly of the National Heart, Lung and Blood Institute.

"Heart disease is related to our modern lifestyle: mechanization, cigarette smoking, television and *spectating* at sporting events instead of participating," said Arthur S. Leon, M.D., from the School of Public Health at the University of Minnesota in Minneapolis. Dr. Leon also said that "endurance-type exercise improves the efficiency of the cardiovascular system." He cited autopsy studies that demonstrate that endurance athletes and physically active people have larger arteries supplying blood to the heart.

For details on the direct benefits of exercise to the heart and blood system, we'll turn to studies of the effects of a specific form of exercise—something we've all taken for granted since early childhood.

Walk, Don't Run, for Your Life

Speak of exercise, and jogging is one of the first activities that come to mind. But jogging is not the only—or even the best—way for many of us to exercise. For each time your foot hits the ground, the 26 bones and 19 muscles in your foot are subjected to shock waves that are transmitted from the heel up through the ankle, calf, knee, thigh, hip and back. The longer and harder you run, the more shock impacts you receive. For those who are a bit out of shape or overweight, repeated shock vibrations can throw the vertebrae out of alignment, thus raising the potential for lower back problems and sciatica.

Walking, however, is much more natural than jogging, and is every bit as much of a boon to health, without the problems inherent in jogging.

One of the doctors involved in bringing forth exciting new research on walking is Dan Streja, M.D., a Canoga Park, California, endocrinologist. "Metabolically speaking," Dr. Streja told us, "walking is as good as jogging. To favorably alter cholesterol, to lower sugar, insulin and triglycerides, and to lose weight, walking will do it. I expect it would lower blood pressure as well."

Along with David Mymin, M.D., of the University of Manitoba in Canada, Dr. Streja has published results of a study in which 32 men, 35 to 68 years old, all with heart disease, were put on a program of walking, working up to slow jogging if they could manage it. But in fact, the average speed of the participants was less than four miles an hour at the beginning of the 13-week program, and just slightly over four miles per hour at the conclusion. Which means that the average speed was no faster than a businesslike walking gait, about as fast as you'd be walking on a cold day. There were only an average of three sessions per week, and the average distance walked at each session was slightly less than 1¾ miles. Yet despite this relatively modest degree of effort, some very impressive results were obtained.

Most importantly, perhaps, there was a very promising change in cholesterol levels. Specifically, there was an increase in the fraction of cholesterol known as HDL. Generally speaking, the higher the HDL, the less chance there is of a heart attack. And in fact, there *was* a significant increase in the HDL count of this group of walkers. Previously, it had been known that long-distance runners and other extremely active types had elevated HDL counts, but this was one of the first times anyone had demonstrated the beneficial effect resulting only from walking.

Besides the increase in HDL, there was a *decrease* in circulating insulin levels.

Now most of us don't think about insulin outside the context of diabetes. But the fact is that many Americans have too much of that hormone drifting through their systems, and—to make a long story very short—high insulin levels can help bring on both diabetes *and* heart disease. Pretty serious stuff. Yet the walkers in the program described enjoyed a very significant decrease in plasma insulin (*Journal of the American Medical Association,* November 16, 1979).

Dr. Mymin further explained that the increase in valuable HDL is "proportional to the strenuousness of the activity. But you don't have to be an athlete to get benefits. *Any* increase in your regular amount of exercise will cause an increase in HDL. Going from inactive to moderately active will cause HDL levels to rise. But so will going from moderately active to very active."

Several other investigators have also found that walking does more than expected for the heart. At a conference of the American Heart Association held in Dallas in November, 1978, a very similar walking plan (45 minutes, three times a week) was reported to significantly improve the HDL ratio in both men and women taking part in a ten-week program. Doctors attending that conference were also told that exercise such as walking increases the amount of blood pumped by the heart, and therefore increases the amount of oxygen reaching all the tissues "no matter how old or sedentary the person."

Other doctors point out that even when exercise is not vigorous enough to infuse the body with fresh oxygen, the burden on the heart is still eased significantly. That's because the more you walk, the more your leg muscles become conditioned to hard work and the less oxygen they need from the heart.

Walking has it all over other forms of exercise when it comes to ease and convenience, so people who choose walking as an exercise are more likely to stick with it.

"A study done by the government several years ago showed that approximately half the people surveyed exercise almost daily, and of those, about one-third said they walk for exercise," said one walking advocate we spoke to. "Now that's far more than participated in any other activity—jogging, swimming, whatever."

How Other Forms of Exercise Measure Up

Of course, walking isn't the *only* way to get into shape. There are so many ways to work out—and enjoy it—that you may decide on a different tack. You could even choose a variety of exercises—bicycling and walking in the summer (or jumping rope when it's rainy) and dancing in the winter. Here's a rundown of the most common types of exercise.

JOGGING. If you decide to run or jog for exercise, it's encouraging to know that you don't have to run great distances to benefit. Researchers at Methodist Hospital and Baylor College of Medicine in Houston studied 44 healthy men aged 41 to 61 years. Twenty-two had completed a marathon within the past year and regularly ran more than 30 miles a week. Another 22 men jogged as little as 2 miles a day, three times a week. Both groups were compared to a third group of men who occasionally played golf, played tennis or did calisthenics but were relatively inactive. Both the joggers and marathoners weighed less and had less body fat than the inactive men, and both groups of runners had significantly higher HDL cholesterol levels and lower triglycerides, two signs of a healthy heart. In addition, maximal oxygen uptake—one of the signs of efficient muscle function, endurance and overall cardiorespiratory (heart and lung) fitness—was higher than expected in the runners and, in fact, rivaled that of men 20 years younger.

"A middle-aged man may not, then, have to become a marathon runner in order to obtain [benefits] which indicate a reduction in risk of coronary heart disease," wrote the researchers (*Preventive Medicine,* May, 1981).

To get those benefits, researchers at the Stanford Heart Disease Prevention Program recommend running an average of about a mile a day. They studied 48 middle-aged men who exercised and 31 who did not and found that men who ran 8½ to 12 miles a week had significantly higher HDL cholesterol levels than the nonexercisers (*Employee Health and Fitness,* May, 1981).

BICYCLING is every bit as good as jogging as far as heart and lung capacity and overall fitness is concerned, but without jogging's constant pounding of the feet, arches, knees, hips and back. Researchers at the Human Performance Laboratory at the University of California at Davis compared the physical benefits of bicycling to jogging and tennis in 38 sedentary, middle-aged men. The men were divided into four groups and assigned to either an exercise or a nonexercise group. For 20 weeks, the experimental groups exercised three days a week for 30 minutes a day. Maximal oxygen uptake — remember, a good indicator of cardiorespiratory fitness — improved equally in those who bicycled and those who jogged. In this study, in fact, bicyclists went joggers one better: some of their body fat was replaced by muscle (*Medicine and Science in Sports and Exercise,* Spring, 1980).

And there's good reason to believe that bicycling's benefits carry into old age. Researchers at the Human Performance Laboratory at California State University in Sacramento studied a 70-year-old lifelong cyclist who had completed a 3,400-mile bike trek from California to Canada in just under five weeks. They marveled at his youthful physique, noting that the oxygen uptake of his muscles reached 76 percent that of young racing cyclists. He also carried none of the excess fat customarily associated with aging. In short, his body and his physical abilities were a match for any young endurance athlete. The researchers credit his good shape to early training and a daily workout of 6 miles a day of vigorous cycling (*Medicine and Science in Sport,* June/July, 1977).

Cyclists also seem to live longer and have fewer heart attacks than nonexercisers, according to a study of 282 male members of an over-50 cycling club in Britain. Not only did many of the club's over-70 members cycle once a week or more throughout the year, but the average life expectancy of club members was 79 years — many years above the average for men (*British Medical Journal,* December 24-31, 1977).

SWIMMING. "Swimming is an excellent exercise," James Counsilman, Ph.D., told us. He should know. Besides being a swimming coach at Indiana University, he is the oldest man to swim the English Channel. "It's a workout for the whole body," he said, "the heart, the lungs, the arms, the legs — even the neck."

Dr. Counsilman also told us that swimming is the most popular exercise. "Jogging may seem more popular because it has more visibility in the newspapers and magazines — and there's also been plenty of publicity given to the sore joints and injuries that jogging causes. Those types of injuries are almost eliminated in swimming."

However, it's not swimming itself, but *water* that's kind to your bones and muscles. Stand in water up to your neck, and you're suddenly 90 percent lighter. That means a person weighing 150 pounds would "weigh" only 15 pounds in the water. And the body's lightness in water gives swimming a "superior advantage over other sports," said Allen Richardson, M.D., chairman of the

USA Swimming Sports Medicine Committee. "Swimming is what is called a non-weight-bearing sport," he told us. "This is great for the joints, especially for people with ankle, shoulder or back problems. It doesn't put stress on the joints."

And if you're overweight, the fact that swimming is a non-weight-bearing sport means you won't have to fight gravity at every step to exercise those pounds away. Swimming burns 350 to 400 calories an hour.

And the last (but not the least) reason swimming may be the best exercise is that it gets you fit *fast*. Scientific studies show that you can get into good shape by swimming only twice a week for 15 minutes each time. Of course, "swimming" doesn't mean splashing around in the pool. But it doesn't mean wearing yourself out, either. Swim a lap (about 25 yards or meters) every minute, and you're doing as much for your heart as any jogger.

TENNIS. The benefits of tennis can be considerable—*if* you're good at the game. If not, you'll spend so much time ferreting out missed and poorly hit balls that you'll get only very short bursts of activity—not nearly enough to give your heart, lungs or muscles a real workout. Researchers at the University of California at Davis who compared tennis, bicycling and jogging found only modest benefits among novice tennis players who played tennis for 30 minutes three times a week. But, say the researchers, had the men played longer (and better), tennis probably would have produced fitness gains similar to those of bicycling and jogging (*Medicine and Science in Sports and Exercise*, Spring, 1980).

SQUASH. As with tennis, squash can be as beneficial as running if you play the game well. If you and your partner are skilled enough to keep the ball in motion for more than half the time, playing a series of long, hard-fought rallies, you can increase your heart rate and achieve other benefits produced by running, said David L. Montgomery, Ph.D., an associate professor at McGill University in Montreal who studied squash players (*Physician and Sportsmedicine*, April, 1981).

RACQUETBALL adopts some of the elements of tennis and squash but is a better fitness builder than tennis because it provides a more intense workout. Four-walled courts keep the ball—and the players—in nearly constant motion—enough motion to shed 700 calories an hour. Like tennis, racquetball can be played by two or four people. But because racquetball is easier to learn than tennis and the equipment is less expensive, you may be more likely to take it up as your favorite sport.

ROPE SKIPPING. You can't beat rope skipping for both convenience and time-saving. The equipment is simple and inexpensive and you can do it anywhere, anytime, indoors or out—provided you stay clear of lamps and chandeliers. Jumping rope benefits the heart and circulation, although it's somewhat less beneficial than jogging because it uses fewer muscles.

Don't start out on a strenuous skipping program right away, though. Bud Gretchell, Ph.D., director of physical fitness programs at the Human Performance Laboratory at Ball State University, suggests that a gradual approach to rope skipping is best. "We suggest, as with beginning joggers, that a person first be able to walk briskly for two or three miles before engaging in a [rope] skipping program. Then the key is to progress slowly with alternate bouts of skipping of no longer than 20 to 30 seconds and equal or longer times for rest, to avoid unnecessary discomfort and possible injury" (*Physician and Sportsmedicine*, February, 1980).

DANCING. If you've tried walking, jogging, bicycling, swimming and all the rest but abandoned them because you simply get bored easily, dancing could be the answer for you. Whether you go for square, folk, jazz, rock or belly dancing, moving to the music gets all your muscles working, your blood circulating and your heart and lungs pumping—while you have fun. In addition to all those physical benefits, you'll probably develop more grace and confidence and improve your self-image. Dancing can even perk up a flagging social life!

Exercise at Any Age

The wonderful thing about exercise is that people at *any* age can benefit.

"Age does not necessarily destroy exercise capacity," said Swedish researcher Per-Olaf Astrand, M.D., at a conference at the National Institutes of Health titled "Exercise in the Elderly—Its Role in Prevention of Physical Decline and in Rehabilitation" in 1977. Talking about growing younger, Dr. Astrand said it is possible to move one's capacity back 15 to 25 years by heavy training.

That means, added Bengt Saltin, M.D., from the University of Copenhagen, that "an active, training middle-aged man can have higher capacity than a younger, sedentary one." And in fact, Herbert A. deVries, Ph.D., from the Andrus Gerontology Center at the University of Southern California, reported the trainability of people in their seventies and eighties is *not* significantly different from that of young people.

Moreover, the psychological benefits of exercise for keeping us young are just as real as the physical benefits. Ken Sidney, Ph.D., from Laurentian University in Sudbury, Ontario, Canada, recruited 42 sedentary, overweight older men and women and put them through the paces—vigorous activities like jogging and brisk walking—for three months. At the outset, all conceded that not one of them was any competition for Jack LaLanne or Diana Nyad; after the exercise program, however, most felt far better about themselves. Not only did most people in the study feel they looked better, but they felt less clumsy, tense and anxious, according to psychological tests. All in all, exercise fired their enthusiasm for staying active (*Medicine and Science in Sport*, Winter, 1976).

Yet in spite of all its youth-bestowing powers, most older people shy away from exercise. Dr. Sidney suggested it's because "people are afraid of exertion. Our culture teaches them to expect to slow down and to degenerate as they grow older. A lot of people are embarrassed to exercise in public, too."

"Doctors are prejudiced, too, against older people," said Michael B. Mock, M.D., formerly of the Cardiac Disease Branch of the National Heart, Lung and Blood Institute. "People think they should be relegated to the rocking chair. A doctor's personality and the way he handles a patient can have an effect on the results of treatment. Doctors sometimes just give a drug for this and a drug for that, but they don't ask questions. They just say, 'Take it easy' and 'No going up steps.' That leads to an overmedicated, vegetative person. And it sometimes results in a person ending up in a nursing home instead of taking care of himself—if he had been given some encouragement to be active, he would have been better off."

So keeping our bodies active seems to be just as important today as it was to our ancestors who had to work all day at surviving. As Elsworth R. Buskirk, Ph.D., from the Laboratory for Human Performance Research at Pennsylvania State University, put it, "Man lives to move and moves to live."

After examining all the evidence, it's obvious that exercise can actually tack additional years onto your calendar of life.

PART II

The Life
Extension Diet

Cut the Fat

Jack Sprat had the right idea. Because above a reasonable minimum—at the most, 20 percent of the diet—fat has no place in any plan for a long life. Heart disease, cancer, diabetes, high blood pressure, gallbladder disease and liver disease—not to mention overweight—are *all* encouraged by a high-fat diet.

Hearts "Live Long and Prosper" on a Lean Diet

In addition to taking up residence on our hips, fat also tends to cling to less visible body parts like the blood vessels. It's there that fat does the most to shorten life. High levels of fat (cholesterol and the triglycerides) in the blood leave deposits on the walls of arteries, narrowing these major blood vessels. That buildup of fat on artery walls—called atherosclerosis—is often responsible for a sudden death from heart attack or the lingering disability of a stroke. And it's not such a big jump from the fat on our dinner plates to the fat in our arteries. According to the *New England Journal of Medicine* (June, 1978), six decades of scientific evidence implicate dietary fat as a major factor in atherosclerosis.

But fatty buildup in blood vessels is only one of the problems. Robert I. Lowenberg, M.D., a vascular surgeon from Atlanta, Georgia, says that high levels of fat in the blood also "neutralize the negative charge that separates red blood cells, making them stick together like a stack of wet dishes. In a healthy person, red blood cells float through blood vessels in single file, absorbing oxygen and discharging it to the tissues. When high fat levels make cells stick together," Dr. Lowenberg continued, "a lot of surface is lost for picking up and delivering oxygen. Tissues begin to suffocate. To make matters worse, the clumped blood cells also get jammed at bends in the capillaries."

All that, in one way or another, helps set the stage for heart and circulatory problems such as deep vein thrombosis—many of which are potentially fatal.

In the case of heart disease, some fats are worse than others. The fats in food, to begin with, come in several chemical varieties. *Saturated* fats, in which each atom of carbon carries all the hydrogen it can hold, are most common in meats. *Polyunsaturated* fats, whose carbon atoms have room for more hydrogen, are found more abundantly in vegetables, and in fish and fowl. A large body of research indicates that saturated fats are the ones to watch in guarding against heart disease. Where the diet is rich in these animal fats, statistics say that heart disease is generally a problem.

Some studies have found that merely substituting poly-unsaturated fats for saturated ones can lower the level of cholesterol in the blood, and with it, presumably, the risk of heart disease. In Finland, long-term patients at one mental hospital were given the normal Finnish diet, which is very high in saturated fat sources like eggs and milk products. In another hospital, much of the saturated fat was replaced with polyunsaturated fat. After six years, the diets were switched. Researchers found that when patients received the polyunsaturated-fat diet, their blood cholesterol dropped sharply. What's more, the rate of death from coronary heart disease in the hospital group on the experimental diet fell to half the rate of people eating the saturated-fat diet at the other institution (*Circulation*, January, 1979).

That is because cholesterol in the blood is transported by complexes of fats and proteins called lipoproteins. Low-density lipoproteins (LDL) carry cholesterol *to* the cells, and high-density lipoproteins (HDL) carry cholesterol *away* from the cells. As a result, a high proportion of LDL has come to be associated with a high risk of atherosclerosis, while a high proportion of HDL is associated with a low risk.

Some studies have suggested that a reduction in saturated fats can raise the level of HDL—the valuable cholesterol that apparently resists the buildup of fatty deposits. Also, substituting polyunsaturated for saturated fats can reduce the tendency of the blood to form thrombi, the tiny blood clots that may initiate heart attacks and strokes.

The danger, however, is to see the two kinds of fats, saturated and polyunsaturated, as "bad fats" and "good fats." In fact, the emerging message of much modern nutritional research is the necessity to cut down on all fats—animal and vegetable, saturated and polyunsaturated. That may be necessary, some investigators say, to reduce the risk not only of heart disease, but of cancer, too.

Less Fat Also Means Less Cancer

Some 50 percent of all cancers, researchers speculate, may be related in part to diet. And fat, according to mounting evidence, is the part of the diet that most bears watching. The evidence has been convincing enough to lead the National Cancer Insitute (NCI) to recommend that Americans consume less fat (among other dietary modifications) to lessen the danger of cancer. And that very definitely includes margarine and corn oil as well as steak and butter.

As in the case of heart disease, what aroused investigators' suspicions was the striking correlation between the amount of fat eaten by various peoples and their susceptibility to certain cancers.

"There exists a worldwide correlation between bowel cancer and fat consumption." wrote Gio B. Gori, Ph.D., formerly of the NCI. Where fats make up a large part of the diet, as in Scotland, Canada and the United States, bowel cancer is common. Where fats are scarce, so is the disease.

Of particular interest is what happens to people who move from one place to another. America, where the average person gets some 40 percent of his calories from fats, has a high incidence of bowel cancer; Japan, where the intake is only 12 percent, has a low rate. But when Japanese immigrate to America, their susceptibility to bowel cancer tends to become "Americanized," too. The children of these immigrants develop much more bowel cancer than their cousins who stayed in Japan.

How can dietary fats increase the danger of developing bowel cancer? According to one theory, excessive fats promote an increased secretion of the bile acids that aid in their digestion. In the large intestine, bacteria may transform these bile acids into cancer-causing chemicals (carcinogens).

Breast Cancer Strongly Linked to Fat Intake

The association between fat and breast cancer seems even stronger. G. Hems, of the Department of Community Medicine in Aberdeen, Scotland, tabulated the breast cancer rates in 41 counties and related them to local diets.

"It was concluded that variations of breast cancer rates between countries arose predominantly from differences in diet," he wrote in the *British Journal of Cancer* (vol. 37, no. 6, 1978). And one place where the shadow of suspicion fell most heavily was on the consumption of fat. Other studies have confirmed that the disease is less common in poor and developing nations, where rich foods are rarely on the menu, than in the wealthier countries of the West. Like bowel cancer, breast cancer increases among Japanese immigrants who give up their low-fat diet for our high-fat diet. But among Seventh-day Adventists, breast cancer mortality rates are only one-half to two-thirds that of Americans in general. Many members of this religious group are vegetarians, and their saturated fat and cholesterol intake is well below the average.

The link between fat and breast cancer, scientists speculate, may be hormones. Studies have related the development of the disease to abnormal levels of prolactin, estrogens and androgens: the production of these hormones apparently goes up with fat intake. A high-fat diet may disturb hormone levels and that, according to one scientist, "could impose unnatural burdens" on the cells of breast tissue, with cancer as the result.

Two relatively recent studies graphically demonstrate the relation of hormone levels in the blood and fat levels in the diet. In South Africa, native black women suffer very little from breast cancer, while white women fall prey to the disease much more frequently. Their diets are markedly different: the native diet is vegetarian and very low in fat—less than 20 percent of its total calories are fat—while the whites consume a typical Western diet in which fat provides 40 percent of the calories. Peter Hill, Ph.D., of the American Health Foundation, measured the hormone levels in groups of black and white women in South Africa, and found more significant differences—the black women had lower levels of a number of hormones, including prolactin. He put the black women on a Western diet for periods of six weeks to two months, and then measured their hormone levels again. He found that the proportions of various hormones had changed substantially: they began to resemble the "hormone profile" of white women. And these new hormone levels—including the rise in prolactin—are ones that have been associated with increased rates of breast cancer (*Federation Proceedings*, abstract no. 3357, March 1, 1979).

Dr. Hill conducted a similar study of South African and North American men. Vegetarian, black South African men have a far lower rate of prostate cancer than North American men, and their diet has about half the fat of the one consumed in America.

In testing their urine, Dr. Hill found that the South Africans excrete considerably less androgens and estrogens than their American counterparts.

For three weeks, Dr. Hill had his subjects switch diets. The Americans ate low-fat, vegetarian food, and the Africans ate rich American fare. Even in this short time, he found a change in diet meant a switch in hormone profiles, too. There was a marked increase in androgen and estrogen excretion among the Africans, while the amount of hormones excreted by the Americans decreased to the point where it resembled the levels of the low-risk group.

It is important to remember that in these studies of diet and cancer, what is generally measured is *total* fat intake. In other words, while replacing saturated with polyunsaturated fats may cut down the risk of heart disease, the substitution seems to offer no protection against cancer.

Beware of Partially Hydrogenated Fats

Some researchers suggest that even polyunsaturated fats may be dangerous where cancer is concerned. In a number of studies, animals fed polyunsaturated fats developed more tumors than those fed saturated fats. And when researchers at the University of Maryland compared human diets with cancer rates, they found a strong association between cancer and vegetable fats.

Those statistics point to one kind of fat, in particular, as a danger—fat containing *trans* fatty acids. *Trans* fatty acids don't occur naturally in vegetables but are produced when polyunsaturated oils are partially hydrogenated, when they are processed with hydrogen to make them more solid or to give them a longer shelf life. Many kinds of margarine, salad oil, mayonnaise and snack foods contain significant amounts of these substances. Quite possibly, researchers speculate, these unnatural *trans* fatty acids alter cell membranes, allowing carcinogens to pass through more easily. People who are trying to reduce their risk of heart disease by substituting margarine and corn oil for butter and animal fat should avoid products labeled "partially hydrogenated."

Fish Oil Does Your Heart Good

If there's one kind of fat you *should* include in your diet, it's fish oil.

"Fish oil contains certain substances that may inhibit the biochemical processes that may lead to stroke and heart attack," said a researcher from the University of Illinois Medical Center. "Thanks to research on fish oil, we are learning more precisely how those processes work and how they can be altered."

Interest in the relationship of fish oil to cardiovascular disease began with findings about obscure tribes of Greenland Eskimos. Those tribes eat a high-fat, high-cholesterol diet—a diet that most evidence says should promote atherosclerosis. Yet among the Eskimos, atherosclerosis and its attendant evils, stroke and heart disease, are rare. What researchers pursuing the dietary causes of those diseases wanted to know was, how could that be?

Noting that the main source of fat in the Eskimo diet is fish, scientists studied the fatty acids found in those animals. Danish scientists observed that fish fats are unique in that they contain relatively high amounts of omega-3 fatty acids (one of the two main classes of polyunsaturated fats). But what was even more significant, they discovered that omega-3 fatty acids reduce the production of a substance that causes blood cells to stick together, a condition that may lead to blocked arteries and eventual stroke or heart attack. The omega-3 fatty acids actually seem to neutralize the bad effects of other fats. If Eskimo arteries are clearer and more supple than those of the average North American, it might be because of the fish Eskimos eat.

"Unfortunately, the average North American diet seldom contains foods rich in these omega-3 fatty acids," said William Harris, Ph.D., a research fellow in nutrition at University of Oregon Health Sciences Center. "Virtually no omega-3 fatty acids are found in beef, chicken or any food but fish. The average American diet consists of 40 percent fat. That creates an imbalance of the 'bad' kind of fatty acids which may then be converted by cellular metabolism into substances that lead to preconditions for stroke and heart attack," Dr. Harris said.

Whisks Away Blood Fats

Would normal Americans who changed to an Eskimo diet enjoy the same benefits? Dr. Harris and two colleagues set out to determine the probable effect of fish oil on risk factors of heart disease. They recruited ten volunteers, five men and five women. For one month, the ten ate a typical American diet, high in fat but including vegetables and fruit. Then tests were done to determine their blood chemistries. The next month, the volunteers switched to the second diet, identical to the first except that its fat came from salmon meat and salmon oil. The blood chemistry tests were again performed, and the results were compared with those following the first diet.

"Our study was designed to answer two questions," Dr. Harris explained. "First, does fish oil in the diet reduce levels of blood fats, such as cholesterol and triglycerides, and thus conceivably help prevent heart disease? Second, does dietary fish oil make blood platelets less sticky and thus reduce the tendency to form blood clots?"

High levels of cholesterol or triglycerides are possible warning signs of coronary trouble. "After a month on the salmon diet," said Dr. Harris, "the average blood cholesterol level went down 17 percent, a moderate decrease. But triglyceride levels dropped 40 percent, which is exciting. There's something unique about the effect of fish oil on triglyceride metabolism. Polyunsaturated vegetable oils will lower cholesterol levels, too, but they don't do much to triglyceride levels."

In order to find out why the blood fat levels fell on the salmon diet, the researchers gave each subject a high-fat breakfast and measured how high the blood fat levels went over the next eight hours. The test showed both how fast the fat was absorbed into the blood and how rapidly it was removed. The doctors found that the blood fat levels after eating saturated fat were higher than after the salmon-fat meal. In other words, salmon fat was either absorbed more slowly or (more likely) it was cleared from the blood more rapidly. That appears to be another unique effect of fish oils.

A Trim-the-Fat Diet

What it all boils down to is, the less fat the better. What's more, we should lean toward fish and vegetable oils for what lubrication we *do* need. And low-fat eating is not difficult, once we follow a few basic principles:

■ Eat fruits, vegetables and whole grains. There is little fat in fruits and vegetables (with the exception of avocados, nuts and coconuts). Whole grains and beans offer a lot of protein without much fat. (See table 1.) Another advantage of fruits, vegetables and whole grains is that they are high in fiber, which also helps lower blood fats. (See the chapter, Put Fiber to Work for You.)

■ Cut down on red meats (beef, pork, lamb and veal). Trimming the fat off the roast is a good idea but it's not enough. Most of the fat that finds its way into our bodies—some 60 percent, according to the USDA—is "invisible fat" and likely to be overlooked in trimming. Even after the fatty edge is removed from a T-bone steak, for example, the meat itself harbors a lot of fat—some 40 percent of its calories.

Table 1
FAT CONTENT OF SOME COMMON FOODS

If you're like most Americans, you get 40 percent or more of your calories from fat. To reduce that level, eat more foods from the end of the list, plus plenty of fish for special fatty acids in fish oil.

Food	% Calories from Fat	Portion	Calories	Fat (grams)
Coconut	92	¼ cup	112	11.0
Avocado	90	½	188	18.5
Hot dog	82	1	184	17.0
Bacon	79	2 thick slices	143	12.5
Cheddar cheese	74	2 ounces	228	19.0
Steak, sirloin, broiled	74	3 ounces	329	27.0
Soup, cream of mushroom	67	1 cup	135	10.0
Egg, poached	63	1	79	6.0
Milk chocolate	56	1 ounce	145	9.0
Salmon, Atlantic	56	3 ounces	229	14.0
Cookies, chocolate chip	53	4 medium	205	12.0
Milk, whole	49	1 cup	150	8.0
Ice cream	48	1 cup	270	14.0
Potatoes, french-fried	43	10	137	6.6
Pie, apple	39	½ of a 9-inch pie	345	15.0
Milk, low-fat	38	1 cup	120	5.0
Tuna, canned in oil, drained	38	3 ounces	166	7.0
Beef, flank steak (100% lean)	33	3 ounces	167	6.2
Pizza	25	⅛ of a 12-inch pie	145	4.0
Yogurt, low-fat	22	1 cup	144	4.0
Chicken, white meat, roasted	19	3 ounces	142	3.0
Pork and beans, canned with tomato sauce	19	½ cup	156	3.3

(continued)

Table 1 — continued

Food	% Calories from Fat	Portion	Calories	Fat (grams)
Buttermilk	18	1 cup	100	2.0
Cottage cheese, low-fat	18	½ cup	101	2.0
Oatmeal	14	1 cup	130	2.0
Whole wheat bread	12	2 slices	122	1.6
Apple	9	1 medium	80	0.8
Tuna, canned in water	6	4 ounces	144	0.9
Beans, navy	5	½ cup	112	0.6
Milk, skim	5	1 cup	86	0.5
Mung beans, sprouted	5	½ cup	19	0.1
Rice, brown	5	1 cup	232	1.2
Peas, split	4	½ cup	115	0.5
Banana	2	1 medium	101	0.2
Haddock	2	4 ounces	111	0.2
Potato	0.8	1 medium	104	0.1
Broccoli	0	1 cup	40	trace
Lentils	0	½ cup	105	trace

SOURCES: Adapted from
Nutritive Value of American Foods in Common Units, Agriculture Handbook No. 456, by Catherine F. Adams (Washington, D.C.: Agricultural Research Service, U.S. Department of Agriculture, 1975).
Composition of Foods: Dairy and Egg Products, Agriculture Handbook No. 8–1, by Consumer and Food Economics Institute (Washington, D.C.: Agricultural Research Service, U.S. Department of Agriculture, 1976).
Composition of Foods: Poultry Products, Agriculture Handbook No. 8–5, by Consumer and Food Economics Institute (Washington, D.C.: Agricultural Research Service, U.S. Department of Agriculture, 1979).
Composition of Foods: Sausages and Luncheon Meats, Agriculture Handbook No. 8–7, by Consumer and Food Economics Institute (Washington, D.C.: Agricultural Research Service, U.S. Department of Agriculture, 1980).

■ Substitute fish and fowl for red meats. Salmon, tuna, trout, mackerel, shad and bass are all rich in valuable omega-3 fatty acids. (Or fish oil supplements, such as cod-liver oil, may be substituted. A letter writer to the British medical journal, *Lancet* [October 6, 1979] suggests two teaspoons, or ten grams, daily. That amount supplies about ten times the usual intake.)

It's best to buy tuna packed in water, not oil. And remove the fatty skin from chicken and turkey.

- Read labels in order to avoid "hydrogenated" or "partially hydrogenated" fats and oils. Natural peanut butter, made from ground peanuts and nothing else, has no hydrogenated fats.

- When eating out, be wary. Some of the most concentrated sources of fat are found in fast-food restaurants. A meal at McDonald's is nearly 40 percent fat, while a serving of Kentucky Fried Chicken is 55 percent fat. Fried foods in classier eateries aren't any leaner.

- Use low-fat dairy products—cottage cheese, skim or low-fat milk, low-fat yogurt. Two-thirds of the calories in some hard cheeses come from fat. And of course, butter is almost pure fat.

- Avoid processed foods. Many processed foods not only contain a hefty load of fat, but that load is often partially hydrogenated and full of *trans* fatty acids. Know exactly what goes into your food.

Cutting down on total fats will also have some important but indirect health benefits. Since fats—animal and vegetable alike—are the most concentrated sources of calories (they have twice the calories, gram for gram, of carbohydrates or protein), a cut in fat intake can produce weight loss. And weight control apparently reduces the risk of both cancer and heart disease. In the bargain, you'll also help protect yourself against a host of other ills, including diabetes, high blood pressure, gallbladder problems and liver disease.

Put Fiber to Work for You

CHAPTER 4

The discovery of the value of food fiber may well do for our generation what the discovery of vitamins did for an earlier generation. It could spark a health revolution, because fiber fights for our lives in many ways.

Fiber is the material in whole grain, beans, potatoes, corn and a wide variety of other fruits and vegetables, that passes through the digestive system untouched. We've all heard since childhood that "roughage"—an earlier name for fiber—is nature's protection against constipation and other problems in the lower end of the digestive system. So how can stuff destined for disposal help preserve our well-being?

Researchers are discovering that an amazingly large number of the so-called "normal" health problems of aging—some of them actually life-*shortening*—can be aggravated by too little fiber in the diet. Putting more fiber under our belts may help avert even the most deadly of these disorders: heart disease, high blood pressure, diabetes and some common forms of cancer.

For example:

■ Fiber helps control weight. Carrying around extra pounds can lop years off our lives. But when we eat a diet rich in fiber, we feel full sooner, eat less and gain less weight.

■ Fiber cuts down fat absorption from food during digestion.

■ Fiber lowers the levels of certain fats (cholesterol and the triglycerides) in the blood, fats which have been strongly linked to heart disease.

■ Fiber seems to help keep blood pressure down.

■ Fiber may help diabetics—and other people—by reducing the body's need for insulin.

■ Fiber discourages bowel cancer from developing because its bulk dilutes cancer-causing substances (carcinogens) in the large intestine and pushes them—along with everything else—through faster.

All those actions, in one way or another, help increase chances of a longer life.

Fiber Scrubs Out Blood Fats

As we mentioned in an earlier chapter, fatty buildup on artery walls is murder on the heart, but, fortunately, fiber "scrubs" away the lethal debris. A U.S. government scientist reported in 1978 that hard red spring wheat and corn bran (part of the whole kernel) both work to up the percentage of high-density lipoproteins (HDL) in the blood. HDL, that fraction of cholesterol now believed to protect the heart, probably does so by helping remove other evil cholesterol relatives from the blood before they can build up on artery walls. As a bonus, the wheat caused a decrease in low-density lipoproteins (LDL)—a decrease which is also considered good—plus a 17 percent decrease in total cholesterol, another good sign. Juan Munoz, M.D., formerly with the Human Nutrition Laboratory in the USDA, also said that wheat and corn, as well as a number of other sources of fiber, reduced triglycerides, another form of blood fat, by about 15 percent.

One medical scientist has reported finding actual improvement in the clinical signs of heart disease in patients taking supplementary fiber. Renzo Romanelli, M.D., professor of gerontology and geriatrics at the University of Pisa in Italy, reported to a 1978 conference of the International College of Surgeons that a number of heart patients taking wheat bran daily suffered fewer angina attacks. In 5 patients over 70 years of age, Dr. Romanelli said, tests also showed an improvement in cardiac efficiency, and fewer EKG (electrocardiogram) signs that the heart muscle was being denied oxygen. In 14 patients between 72 and 94 years of age, he added, there was complete disappearance of a particular kind of circulatory inefficiency which commonly occurs during straining at stool. The professor explained that with a low-fiber diet, constipation and the need to strain often result. High pressures can build up in the colon during elimination and this condition demands more work from the heart. Bran puts an end to that cycle. Fiber, Dr. Romanelli told the assembled surgeons, is so important that its inclusion in the daily diet should be a part of all preventive medicine.

Pectin, a kind of fiber found in apples and in the white rind of oranges, is another natural substance that can help lower cholesterol. A review of medical journals by A. Stewart Truswell, M.D., of

Queen Elizabeth College, London University, England, points out that there have been at least seven recent reports on pectin and cholesterol and "all found a significant reduction of. . .cholesterol" when this fiber was added to patients' diets.

When Fiber Goes Up, Blood Pressure Comes Down

Blood pressure—the force with which blood courses through the arteries—can go up for a variety of reasons, some clear and some unclear. But each step above a normal blood pressure (about 140/90 or lower, depending on one's age, sex, race and medical history) increases our chances of death from heart attack, stroke or kidney failure. Turning that around, any means we can use to bring the blood pressure down will increase our chances for a longer life. Fiber's role in lowering blood pressure was not really addressed until 1978. Then, a group of scientists with the USDA and the University of Maryland discovered, almost by accident, that it tends to go down when dietary fiber goes up. The study was reported by June L. Kelsay, Ph.D., and several colleagues, who had hoped to discover the effect of moderate amounts of fiber from fruits and vegetables on the absorption of nutrients. The researchers placed a group of volunteers on two diets: first a low-fiber diet and then some high-fiber fare. Neither diet was remarkably different from what most people already eat. The doctors didn't learn much about nutrient absorption, but they found that the average blood pressure of all 12 men in the study went down slightly with the high-fiber diet. It wasn't a statistically significant amount in all the subjects, but there was an important change in 6 of the 12, 6 men whose diastolic pressure had been higher than 80. In this group, the average blood pressure fell from 123/88 on the low-fiber diet to 118/78 on the high-fiber diet. (The first number of the two is the systolic pressure, the highest pressure reached, just after the heart contracts. The second number is the diastolic pressure, the lowest pressure reached, when the heart is at rest between beats.)

Although it's true that only six men showed improvement, a drop of ten points in diastolic blood pressure can have very real health benefits, according to the researchers (*American Journal of Clinical Nutrition*, July, 1978).

Fiber Heads Off Diabetes

Diabetes is the third leading cause of death in our country, accounting for 300,000 to 350,000 lives lost each year. The toll climbs even higher when we consider the deadly complications of diabetes. In half of the deaths from heart attack and three-quarters of those from stroke each year, diabetes is the underlying cause of the fatal circulatory disease. In fact, heart disease is the major cause of death among diabetics.

Diabetes is not at all rare. The American Diabetes Association estimates that 1 out of every 20 Americans will be diabetic sometime in the course of a lifetime. And the older we get, the more susceptible we become. Some 40 to 60 percent of people in their eighties suffer from diabetes.

The disease represents a failure of the body's ability to use carbohydrates. When we eat carbohydrates, glucose (or blood sugar) is produced for immediate use or stored for later. Stored glucose is released into the bloodstream whenever we need an energy boost. Insulin, a hormone produced by the pancreas, regulates the level of glucose in the blood. In diabetes, the insulin cannot hold down glucose levels, and diabetics often need injections of outside insulin to do the job.

But fiber can change all that. Scientists are finding that certain diabetic patients can decrease or even eliminate their use of insulin. And some of the most encouraging successes have been achieved using a high-carbohydrate, high-fiber diet.

James Anderson, M.D., of the University of Kentucky, has been working with high-fiber diets for some years. Studies with thin diabetic men showed that the diet not only reduces the need for insulin but also lowers the levels of fats in the blood, fats that have been linked to heart disease. "These short-term improvements have been sustained for up to five years in lean patients who follow high-fiber. . .diets," Dr. Anderson reported in 1979.

Dr. Anderson's most recent study involved diabetic people with weight problems. Obese diabetics, like thin diabetics, were able to lower both their use of insulin and the level of dangerous fats in their blood by eating a high-fiber diet (*Obesity and Bariatric Medicine*), July/August, 1980).

Note: *If you are currently under treatment for diabetes, it is important that you consult your doctor before contemplating a dietary change of any kind.*

Fiber Wards Off Cancer

Along with too much fat in the diet (which we discussed in chapter 3), too little fiber can also pave the way for certain forms of cancer. The growth of colon cancer seems to start with chemical substances called bile acids, which are formed in the liver and secreted into the bile fluid.

"Animals on a high-fat diet given a colon carcinogen develop more colon cancers than animals on a low-fat diet" reported John H. Weisburger, Ph.D., and Ernst L. Wynder, M.D., of the American Health Foundation in Valhalla, New York. "Such animals excrete larger amounts of bile acids, as do human volunteers and colon cancer patients on a high-fiber diet. A number of lines of evidence indicate that bile acids act as promoters [of the malignancy]."

But fiber evidently can block that promotion. In a paper presented at the National Symposium on Colorectal Cancer in New York City in 1980, Dr. Weisburger and Dr. Wynder pointed out that "several types of fiber inhibit colon carcinogenesis in rats, by diluting bile acids in intestinal bulk. . . ." What's more, they said that the same protective mechanism operates in man.

"A high-risk population consumes high levels of dietary fat, which translates into high levels of intestinal bile acids," the doctors reported. "Intake of a fiber such as wheat bran produces larger intestinal bulk, which serves to dilute the effect of bile acids as cancer promoters." (Fiber absorbs and holds on to liquids like a sponge soaks up water. The more fiber we eat, the bigger the "sponge.") Dr. Weisburger and Dr. Wynder suggest that cutting fat intake and boosting fiber can help prevent colon cancer in the population at large. That diet might even be able to prevent its recurrence in people who have already undergone surgery for removal of a malignancy, they added.

These recommendations were echoed by another American Health Foundation representative at the New York symposium, Bandaru S. Reddy, D.V.M., Ph.D. "In the United States, large bowel cancer ranks highest in incidence of all types of cancer, except for easily detectable and curable skin cancer," said Dr. Reddy, who heads the nutrition division of the Naylor Dana Institute for Disease Prevention in Valhalla, New York. He noted that the lowest rates of colon cancer occur in Africa, Asia and South America where people eat cereal- and vegetable-based diets that are high in fiber and low in fatty foods like meat. Two exceptions that prove the rule are Argentina and Uruguay, where beef is more widely available than elsewhere in South America and, consequently, where bowel cancer rates are high.

Dr. Reddy and several associates compared middle-aged, healthy men living in Kuopio, Finland, who were traditionally at low-risk for colon cancer, with a high-risk group in New York City. They found some interesting differences. Although both groups ate a diet that was relatively high in fat, the men in Finland also ate large amounts of fiber, while those in New York did not

(*Cancer Letters*, April, 1978). "The people in Finland consumed more than twice as much fiber as the people in New York did," Dr. Reddy told us. The men in Kuopio ate lots of whole rye bread and whole grain cereals — excellent sources of dietary fiber — and, as a result, they tended to have bulkier stools. In fact, their daily stool output was three times greater than the New York group's. So while the total bile acid production in both groups was the same, the tumor-promoting bile acids were more diluted (and less harmful) in the Finnish group.

Additional evidence of fiber's protective value turned up in a study by the Kaiser-Permanente Medical Care Program and the California State Department of Health. Researchers there examined the diets of 99 colorectal cancer patients and compared them with the diets of 280 people without gastrointestinal cancer. They found that the patients with colon cancer ate fewer high-fiber foods than the control group. To be specific, the people with colon cancer ate less of such foods as oatmeal, bran cereal, corn bread, lima beans, black-eyed peas, turnips, sweet potatoes and cabbage (*American Journal of Epidemiology*, February, 1979).

An even more direct link between fiber and cancer protection — at least in animals — was demonstrated by researchers at the McGill University Surgical Clinic and Montreal General Hospital. They found that when laboratory rats were injected with a tumor-causing chemical, those that also got fiber developed less colon cancer than those that got none. And the more fiber the animals ate, the less likely they were to develop cancer (*Lancet*, September 9, 1978).

Research results like that have caused Dr. Reddy to conclude, "We think the time has come to make dietary recommendations to the public at large." When we asked him what kind of recommendations he had in mind, he told us, "Personally, I recommend that people reduce their total intake of dietary fat, and I mean both animal and vegetable fat. I also suggest that they increase their intake of dietary fiber. Actually, it's all interrelated — so doing the one thing almost automatically helps to accomplish the other. When you examine the diets of people in various countries around the world, you find that those high in fat are naturally low in fiber and vice versa. Our findings in Kuopio, Finland, were the exception to that rule. There, the diet was actually high in both fat and fiber." And apparently fiber's protective effect prevails.

The richest source of food fiber, bar none, is miller's bran, which is that part of wheat removed during the manufacture of white flour. Miller's bran is 44 percent fiber, according to figures cited by the British fiber authority Denis P. Burkitt, M.D., and

Table 2
SELECTED DIETARY SOURCES
OF FIBER

Food	Portion	Total Fiber (grams)
Sweet potato	1 medium	7.2
Apple	1 medium	6.8
Spinach, cooked	½ cup	5.7
Whole wheat bread	2 slices	5.4
Potato	1 medium	5.3
Almonds	¼ cup	5.1
Beans, kidney	½ cup	4.5
Beans, white	½ cup	4.2
Corn	½ cup	3.9
Peas, raw	½ cup	3.8
Blackberries	½ cup	3.7
Lentils	½ cup	3.7
Pear	1 medium	3.5
Plums	3 medium	3.5
Banana	1 medium	3.2
Beans, pinto	½ cup	3.1
Peanuts	¼ cup	3.0
Orange	1 medium	2.9
Rolled oats	½ cup	2.8
Coconut, shredded	¼ cup	2.7
Broccoli	½ cup	2.6
Raisins	¼ cup	2.5
Zucchini	½ cup	2.5
Barley	½ cup	2.2
Carrots, cooked	½ cup	2.2
Squash, summer	½ cup	2.2
Apricots	3 medium	2.0
Brussels sprouts	½ cup	1.8
Tangerine	1 medium	1.8
Beans, string	½ cup	1.7
Onions, cooked	½ cup	1.6
Pineapple	1 cup	1.6
Walnuts	¼ cup	1.6
Beets	½ cup	1.5
Strawberries	½ cup	1.5
Beans, lima; dried, cooked	½ cup	1.4
Kale, cooked	½ cup	1.4
Tomato	1 medium	1.4

Food	Portion	Total Fiber (grams)
Brown rice	½ cup	1.3
Asparagus, chopped	½ cup	1.2
Celery	1 stalk	1.2
Cabbage, raw, shredded	½ cup	1.1
Cucumbers, sliced	½ cup	1.1
Peaches	1 medium	1.0
Cauliflower, cooked	½ cup	0.9
Cherries	½ cup	0.8

SOURCES: Adapted from
"Composition of Foods Commonly Used in Diets for Persons with Diabetes," by James W. Anderson, M.D., *Diabetes Care*, September/October, 1978.
McCance and Widdowson's The Composition of Foods, by A. A. Paul and D. A. T. Southgate (Elsevier/North-Holland Biomedical, 1978).

Peter Meisner, M.D. (*Geriatrics*, February, 1979). Next come certain fiber-rich breakfast cereals, which are up to 25 percent fiber, and minimally processed cereals and whole grain bread. Peas and beans contain a valuable 7 to 8 percent, and root vegetables like potatoes and carrots are nearly 6 percent fiber— still a useful amount. Processing, you should know, often strips most of the fiber from naturally fiber-rich foods. Ounce for ounce, a baked potato, for instance, has three times more fiber than canned potatoes, two times more fiber than dehydrated potatoes, and 50 percent more fiber than frozen mashed potatoes. See table 2 for a more detailed list of dietary sources of fiber.

Added bonus: Certain high-fiber foods offer even more protection against cancer. Brussels sprouts, cabbage, cauliflower and broccoli contain compounds that can soften the effects of certain environmental carcinogens. And legumes like soybeans and lima beans contain substances called "protease inhibitors," which, reports Gio B. Gori, Ph.D., formerly with the National Cancer Institute, have an antitumor effect. Men who eat a lot of green and yellow leafy vegetables, for instance, seem to get less prostate and colon cancer. Because people have eaten a diet rich in fiber since our very beginning, it makes sense that our recent discovery of fiber's benefits will one day mean as much to our well-being as the earlier discovery of vitamins. And it's nice to learn, once again, that older, simpler things can still solve some of the problems of our newer, more complicated world.

Hold the Salt and Sugar

CHAPTER 5

Salt and sugar are by far our most ubiquitous food additives. They're *everywhere*. And while we're used to headlines that question the safety of other, more horrible-sounding additives, it's probably true that salt and sugar together do more to shorten our lives than all the others combined. To be blunt, salt and sugar, except in tiny amounts, are two things we can live without; in fact, we could probably live *longer* without them.

First, consider that one in every five adults in the United States has high blood pressure, and it *doubles* his or her chances of stroke or heart attack.

Then consider:

■ Salt encourages a rise in blood pressure (also called hypertension) in susceptible—often unwittingly susceptible—people.

■ To make matters worse, sugar in the diet seems to *enhance* that effect of salt.

■ Sugar also contributes to overweight, diabetes and heart disease, all life-shortening conditions.

Yet statistics tell us that the average American—who would deny that he's excessive in anything—eats about 9 pounds of salt and 90 pounds of sugar a year. So it seems a lot of people are salting and sugaring their way to an early grave. Cutting down on salt and sugar—and the sooner, the better—can help change that sweet and deadly course.

Pass Up High Blood Pressure by Passing Up Salt

Blood pressure is the force at which the blood travels
through our arteries after a pump from the heart. There are several

factors that determine that force—body weight, stress and smoking habits, to name a few. But sodium, a main constituent of salt, is an important factor here, too, because it affects blood volume and pressure in two ways, one good and one bad. Working with the kidneys, sodium keeps us from losing too much fluid—from dehydrating. That's good. Too much sodium, however, causes the body to retain fluid, which increases the volume of blood to be pumped through the body. That swell in volume demands a more vigorous thrust by the heart and produces a greater push against artery walls. Blood pressure mounts, and that's bad.

At the same time, sodium seems to prompt the smooth muscles around the smallest arteries to narrow, increasing their resistance to blood flow. Sodium may also act here by accidentally stimulating angiotensin, a hormone that affects the kidneys during periods of stress and causes the heart to beat faster and the blood vessels to contract.

As a result of those actions, sodium promotes high blood pressure in millions of people who happen to be especially sensitive to its effects. Heredity gives some clue to individual vulnerability. If one of your parents has high blood pressure, your chances of developing it are a little better than one in two. If both your parents have it, chances are about three in four that you will, too. But you or your parents can have high blood pressure for years and not know it. High blood pressure has no outward symptoms until it's dangerously high, and milder cases may be detected only in routine medical exams. And while high blood pressure may not show up until advancing years, it can start in infancy.

As a means of reducing high blood pressure, cutbacks in sodium certainly pose no threat to either health or well-being. We need only a tiny amount of sodium. Half a gram (500 milligrams) a day or less is considered sufficient. Yet the average North American gets about four or five grams (4,000 to 5,000 milligrams) of sodium each day. Some of it is naturally present in food. More is added during commercial food processing, and another big dose comes from salt added in the kitchen and at the table. Just one teaspoon of salt contains a shade more than two grams (2,000 milligrams) of sodium.

Obviously, then, cutting down on our use of the saltshaker and eating less commercially prepared food are the two most important steps toward preventing salt-activated high blood pressure. The American Heart Association—and many doctors—wisely recommend moderate salt intake for everyone, infants and children included. Most recently, food manufacturers have been urged to cut down on the amount of salt (or other sodium compounds) they add to packaged foods.

Potassium Helps Flush Out Sodium

There's an important corollary to all that: When sodium intake goes up, potassium intake goes down, largely because the same processing methods that add sodium to foods—the canning and freezing of vegetables, for instance—can deplete potassium by half. And these losses are critical, because adequate potassium intake seems to protect against salt-induced high blood pressure.

Two recent studies, conducted at the London Hospital Medical Center, show just that. In the first study, a group of 16 people with mild hypertension and a group with normal blood pressure received two different diets, each for a period of 12 weeks. During the first 12 weeks, both groups ate a normal diet and took sodium tablets. During the second period, their normal diets were supplemented with potassium, and they were told to avoid salty foods and the use of salt while cooking or at the table.

The high-sodium diet produced a slow rise in blood pressure in both groups. But while eating the high-potassium/low-sodium diet, both systolic and diastolic blood pressure (top and bottom numbers in the blood pressure ratio) fell sharply and significantly in the people with high blood pressure. (People with normal blood pressure experienced small, meaningless rises in blood pressure on that diet.)

A month after the study ended and the subjects had returned to their regular eating habits, both groups were tested a final time. The hypertensives' blood pressure had shot back up again. The researchers concluded that the startling drop in their blood pressure during the high-potassium/low-sodium diet had come from the increase in potassium. This seemed true because the first diet included a small rise in sodium but a large decline in potassium. They added, however, that "the mechanism of this depressor [pressure-lowering] response remains unknown" (*Lancet*, January 10, 1981).

Potassium is most plentiful in fresh fruits, vegetables and lean meats. Potatoes, avocados, blackstrap molasses, cooked lima beans, sardines, flounder, orange juice, winter squash, tomatoes, bananas, milk, cod, and beef liver each contain more than 300 milligrams of potassium per serving. (The minimum daily need for potassium is estimated to be 2,500 milligrams.)

Life Can Be Sweeter and Longer without Sugar

By now, everyone knows that sugar offers plenty of thigh-padding calories but no nutrition. No vitamins, no minerals, no fiber. But there's another error to chalk up against the white stuff: It can increase the threat that salt adds to the diet by raising blood pressure. Sugar coupled with salt plus fat adds up to triple trouble for your heart and arteries.

Blood Pressure Soars with Salt Plus Sugar

Several years ago, Richard A. Ahrens, Ph.D., a professor of food and nutrition at the University of Maryland, discovered the combined effect of salt and sugar on blood pressure. Two groups of rats were put on experimental diets. During the test period, both groups were maintained on salted water, and one was given sugar as a carbohydrate bonus while the other got starch. At the end of the study, the body tissues of those on the sugar regimen were significantly more waterlogged (*Sweeteners: Issues and Uncertainties*, National Academy of Sciences, 1975). That got Dr. Ahrens wondering if sugar might increase salt's ability to bring on high blood pressure. He didn't have to wait long to find out.

Christine G. Beebe, Rachel Schemmel, Ph.D., and Olaf Mickelsen, Ph.D., while at Michigan State University, were preparing a paper on that very topic. The three researchers divided 64 rats into four groups and fed each group a special diet: one got a total grain diet, another a high-sugar diet, still another a high-starch diet, and the last got a high-fat diet. For the first ten weeks the rats were given distilled water to drink, and for the next ten weeks they got salted water.

After the first ten-week period, all the rats had normal systolic blood pressure readings. But those fed sugar had significantly higher blood pressures than those on the grain diet (127 as opposed to 109).

After switching to the salt water, however, it was another story. All the rats except those on the grain rations had systolic blood pressure readings exceeding 140, a figure called hypertension by many investigators. Yet, at the close of the study, only the blood pressures of those eating sugar continued to climb, reaching a critically high reading of 170.

The high death rate during this study prompted the researchers to conduct a second test. This time they decreased the salt content in the diets. But still the sugar menace reared its ugly head. After 18 weeks, the rats fed the high-sugar diet were again classified as hypertensive.

Those researchers also cite other studies that give the "thumbs down" to sugar. One discovered that rats fed a high-sugar diet develop higher blood pressures at younger ages. Another noted decreased life spans in rats when their sugar consumption was increased from 15 to 30 percent of their diet. And still others cite kidney problems as dangerous side effects of a diet laden with sugar (*Proceedings of the Society for Experimental Biology and Medicine*, vol. 151, 1976).

Still more recently an experiment with monkeys helped solidify suspicions about sugar as an accomplice in high blood pressure. Researchers at Louisiana State University Medical School examined the responses of three groups of monkeys to high intakes of salt and sugar. The first group was fed a diet containing no added salt; the second group get a diet with 3 percent salt; and the third group ate a diet containing 3 percent salt plus 38 percent sugar. Those amounts of salt and sugar are high, but they are "within the range of human consumption," according to the researchers.

The doctors found that the monkeys on the salt-plus-sugar diet showed more severe symptoms of high blood pressure than both the other groups. And they concluded their report with this cautiously worded but clear warning: ". . .the synergistic effect of dietary sodium and sucrose [sugar] on the induction of hypertension in this nonhuman primate species has a potentially important bearing on human hypertension" (*American Journal of Clinical Nutrition*, March, 1980).

In other words, what's bad for monkeys is probably bad for people.

Diabetes and Heart Disease Tied to Sugar

High blood pressure aside, sugar also looks bad in relation to diabetes and heart disease. Sheldon Reiser, Ph.D., laboratory chief of the USDA's Carbohydrate Nutrition Laboratory at the Nutrition Institute in Beltsville, Maryland, wanted to find out exactly how sugar contributes to those diseases. Dr. Reiser and his research team convinced 19 volunteers (10 men and 9 women) to take their meals at the Nutrition Institute. All were fed a diet similar to the average American diet in carbohydrate, fat and protein composition. There was just one variation: during the first six weeks, approximately half of the group received 30 percent of their total calories from wheat starch in the form of wafers, while the other half got an equal percentage of their intake from sugar eaten as a cakelike dessert. In the second six-week period the groups exchanged diets and treats. The 30 percent sugar intake was designed to stimulate the effect of a lifetime of sugar consumption in the short period.

Once a week after rising and before eating, the volunteers were asked to roll up their sleeves and give blood for analysis. One interesting finding was that blood levels of sugar and insulin (the hormone necessary for sugar metabolism) were significantly and consistently higher while the volunteers ate the sugar diet than when they followed the starch diet (*Federation Proceedings*, abstract no. 2191, March 1, 1978). According to Dr. Reiser, this indicates that sugar consumption—even in the daily amounts typically consumed by Americans—could be a contributing factor in the development of diabetes later in life.

Refined sugar enters the bloodstream very quickly, Dr. Reiser explained to us. If you load yourself with sugar, your blood sugar levels increase rapidly, triggering a surge of insulin. When this practice is continued on a day-in, day-out basis—as was the case in these six-week trials—insulin insensitivity may result. Eventually you need more insulin to do the same job.

"This is precisely what happens in late-onset diabetes," Dr. Reiser told us. "Hyperinsulinism [high insulin levels in the blood] precedes its onset."

And higher insulin levels can cause more than diabetes in some people. It can become the straw that breaks the camel's back in people prone to heart disease.

"It appears that insulin levels and triglyceride levels have a tendency to rise simultaneously," said the USDA biochemist.

As we've mentioned elsewhere, triglyceride and cholesterol levels are important risk factors for heart disease.

Be a Sugar Sleuth

Cutting out sugar takes cunning. Whisking the sugar bowl off the table doesn't necessarily do the trick. As a food ingredient, sugar is a chameleon. An unbelievable number of prepackaged food items conceal a form of sugar under names like "corn syrup," "corn sweetener," "cane syrup" or similar sugar synonyms. For example, most words that end in "-ose"—sucrose, dextrose, fructose—are actually disguised forms of sugar. As a result, you may be eating more sugar than you realize. In addition to the most obvious items (like sodas, baked goods, desserts and presweetened cereals), baby foods, fruit drinks, salad dressings, soups, ketchup, some canned vegetables and most canned fruits all contain sugar. So read labels before you buy. Better yet, avoid prepackaged foods as much as possible. By doing so, you'll also be avoiding a lot of salt and fat. You heart will appreciate it, and so will your waistline.

A problem, we guess—this combing the supermarket shelves for hidden sugar, salt and fat. But it seems a small expenditure of time and effort (plus, of course, a little taste reeducation) that brings a big dividend—nothing less than an addition of healthy years to our lives.

Supplements for the Best Years of Your Life

CHAPTER **6**

Can taking vitamin supplements help you live longer?

It looks that way.

Of course, good nutrition can't make us live longer than our genes intend, but current views suggest that it can help insure that we live as long as we possibly can, in the very best health possible.

A Classic Study on Nutrition and Long Life

A number of studies imply that a higher than normal intake of vitamin C, to name just one nutrient, appears to lower the chance of death when older people fall ill and to increase their longevity in general. Other studies have shown similar tendencies for other nutrients. What's become the classic study in the field of nutrition and aging, though, is a San Mateo County, California, survey of health and nutrition in 577 people over the age of 50, begun in 1948. Dietary intake of various nutrients was closely measured. Various biochemical tests associated with health and disease (such as blood levels of cholesterol, vitamin C and sugar) were taken. Diseases were recorded. Four years later, Harold D. Chope, M.D., assessed the health of 306 of the original group and turned to the record books to see what role nutrition had played in their aging process.

He found the *people with higher-than-average intakes of vitamins A and C tended to live longer* than those with lower intakes.

How much longer? Quite a bit! Among the people whose intake of vitamin A was less than 5,000 international units (I.U.) a day, the death rate was 13.9 percent. That is, almost 14 percent of their original number had died over the four-year period. For those whose daily intake of vitamin A was 5,000 to 8,000 I.U., the death rate was 6.9 percent. But among those whose daily intake was 8,000 I.U. or more, the death rate was only 4.3 percent.

The data on vitamin C was even more remarkable. Among those whose intake was *less* than 50 milligrams per day, the death rate was 18.5 percent. For those whose daily intake was *over* 50 milligrams, the death rate was only 4.5 percent.

Besides making a big difference in how long those Californians lived, nutrition also made a big difference in what doctors call "morbidity"—illness and suffering. Dr. Chope wrote in the report of his study that in many and varied ways, low intake of specific nutrients was associated with disease of certain body systems, and higher than average intake of those nutrients was associated with lower occurrence of those diseases (*California Medicine,* November, 1954).

A lot of research has been done since then, both on longevity in general and on the role of nutrition in aging. And while many have suspected that nutrition is a key factor in how fast (or how slowly) we age, exciting new revelations are beginning to show *why* it may be true.

Nutrition and the Prospects for Slower Aging

Some scientists theorize that aging occurs mainly through a process called oxidation. That process, we're told, can be controlled by ordinary nutrients, including vitamins E, C, and A, and the mineral selenium.

To understand that theory, let's look at what happens to butter when it sits in the sun. The heat and light produce a chemical change—oxidation—that turns the fat rancid. In the body, a warm environment and exposure to light produces the same chemical reaction. To a degree, oxidation is necessary for the normal working of the body, but the reaction, when it gets out of hand, can cause problems in the fats found in cell membranes. Oxidation of those fats disrupts the delicate functioning of the membrane and can break it open, killing the cell.

In nature's plan, ordinary substances—antioxidants—exist to retard harmful oxidation. Food manufacturers, for example, have known for some time that adding vitamin E or vitamin C to products can control oxidation (and therefore, rancidity) in food.

Applying that principle to human nutrition, scientists suggest that these same natural antioxidants could protect our own cells from oxidation's damage, and that they might be able to prevent some of the tissue and function breakdown we collectively call aging.

VITAMIN E. Vitamin E appears to be the most promising antioxidant. In 1976, Jeffrey Bland, Ph.D., a chemist at the University of Puget Sound in Washington, found that vitamin E prevented changes in red blood cells that ordinarily occur with old age. As red blood cells age, they often develop a popcornlike shape and are called "budded" cells. Dr. Bland believed that budded cells are the result of oxidation in the cell membrane. Oxidation, he suspected, weakens the membrane until the cell pops out of shape the way a tire tube slips through a slit in the tire.

Sure enough, when Dr. Bland exposed red blood cells to light and oxygen, the optimum conditions for oxidation, he found he could produce budded cells in the laboratory. More importantly, he found that when blood donors were given 600 I.U. of vitamin E a day for ten days before they donated blood, their red blood cells seemed free of the deformity. When cells taken from these people receiving E were exposed to light and oxygen for 16 hours, only a small number lost their normal shape. However, cells from people who were not taking vitamin E were transformed into budded cells by the treatment.

Dr. Bland points out that the 600-I.U. dosage of vitamin E was arbitrarily chosen.His research has since shown that the optimal dose for each individual varies greatly, from 100 to 1,200 I.U. daily.

Denham Harman, M.D., Ph.D., of the University of Nebraska, has been working with antioxidants for over 20 years, and has discovered that a number of them, including vitamin E, can prolong the lives of mice. And there have been reports linking E to longevity of *human* cells. One study found that the life span of human cells in the laboratory was increased 100 percent if the cells were grown in a culture with vitamin E added.

Part of the harmful effect of oxidation may be due to some of its waste products called "free radicals"—out-of-control molecules that seem to be an important factor in the wear and tear associated with aging. Dr. Harman, as the chief proponent of that theory, believes that cancer, heart disease, high blood pressure and senility are all caused, in part, by free radicals. He told us that a diet that includes ample amounts of vitamin E could "lessen the possibility of those health problems occurring." Such a diet, he said, "may reasonably be expected to add five to ten or more years of healthy, productive life to the life span of the average person."

VITAMIN A AND SELENIUM. Nutrients other than vitamin E have also been found to act as antioxidants. Scientists in India have discovered that vitamin A fed to rats can block the oxidation that normally occurs when animal tissue is exposed to air. And when the scientists fed vitamin E along with the A, the antioxidant effect was even stronger (*International Journal of Vitamin and Nutrition Research*, vol. 47, no. 4, 1977).

An enzyme in the body called glutathione peroxidase also protects cell membranes from oxidation. The activity of that enzyme in animals has been shown to be directly related to the amount of selenium in the diet. Zinc and manganese might also be needed for the proper functioning of another antioxidant enzyme, superoxide dismutase.

Vitamin E for Lifelong Immunity

Dr. Harman has also been looking at the effects of antioxidants on the body's defenses against disease. Several years ago he demonstrated that a number of antioxidants, including vitamin E, significantly enhanced the immune responses of mice (*Journal of the American Geriatrics Society*, September, 1977). The evidence suggested that oxidation might disrupt the cells involved in mobilizing the body's defenses.

Other researchers, too, have turned their attention to the possible links between antioxidants, immunity and aging. Ronald R. Watson, Ph.D., of Purdue University, told us, "The immune systems in young children and in older people are less effective than in mature adults. The longer you live, the more severely infections hit you. That's why flu vaccine complications usually develop in young people and older people."

Dr. Watson has been testing the effects of diet on the immune systems of people in nursing homes and on laboratory animals. "Our animal studies are going on continuously," he told us. "We've looked at diets high in vitamin E, high- and low-fat diets, and high- and low-protein diets, to see what changes they produce in the immune system."

Dr. Watson's tests of vitamin E produced the same results as Dr. Harman's. "We found that vitamin E boosted one aspect of the immune response, one important in the body's anticancer defenses, within a week of giving it to the mice." Dr. Watson said it's still unclear whether or not that effect is the result of vitamin E's antioxidant properties.

J. Terrell Hoffeld, D.D.S., Ph.D., is another researcher looking into connections between antioxidants and immunity. A scientist at the National Institute of Dental Research, Dr. Hoffeld is looking for a way to combat periodontal disease, an infectious disease of the gums. In the course of his research, Dr. Hoffeld examined the action of different antioxidants in protecting lymphocytes from oxidation. Lymphocytes are cells that play a central role in the immune system. Dr. Hoffeld found that when antioxidant agents block damage to the lymphocytes of mice, the immune response of those cells goes up (*Federation Proceedings,* March 1, 1980).

"We found that agents that acted at multiple sites were more effective," Dr. Hoffeld told us. "A whole series of biochemical reactions is involved in the initiation of oxidation damage to a cell. If you can block those reactions in the early steps, then you can block the final result more efficiently.

"The most effective agent we found was vitamin E," Dr. Hoffeld told us. "Vitamin E acts everywhere along the chain of steps, and therefore is very effective."

Diet Isn't Enough

"Greater amounts of vitamin E in the diet can help to prevent the cells of our bodies from aging faster than necessary," Dr. Jeffrey Bland told us. He recommends between 100 and 400 I.U. of vitamin E a day to help keep cells young and to protect the whole body from smog, radiation and other types of stress that can produce tissue wear and tear.

Another scientist who studies aging, Johan Bjorksten, Ph.D., says that the Recommended Dietary Allowance (RDA) for vitamin E is the amount "necessary to avert obvious deficiency symptoms, but it is by no means the [best amount] for longevity." He thinks that a daily supplement of 200 to 300 I.U. could extend a person's life span by 5 to 15 years (*Rejuvenation*, April, 1975).

The daily amounts of vitamin E recommended by the scientists we spoke to—anywhere from 100 to 600 I.U.—are much higher than levels found in even the most natural and wholesome diet. The amount of vitamin E suggested by Dr. Bland is about 35 *times* the RDA set by the government. But, as one study has shown, there are no harmful effects from taking as much as 800 I.U. a day for many years, and so you can apparently use vitamin E with confidence (*American Journal of Clinical Nutrition*, December, 1975).

Of course, even if you take a vitamin E supplement, you should still get as much vitamin E from your food as you can. And that's simple to do—avoid processed and refined foods. Canned and frozen foods lose up to 65 percent of their vitamin E in processing. Grains are a good source of the vitamin, at least until they're milled. Corn, in becoming corn flakes, loses 98 percent of its vitamin E. Whole wheat bread has seven times more vitamin E than white bread, and brown rice has six times more than white rice. Nuts, another good source, lose up to 80 percent of their vitamin E when they're roasted. Oils, too, provide plenty of vitamin E—unless they've been partially hydrogenated. For the most vitamin E, eat whole foods.

Calcium for Bones That Last as Long as You Do

Oxidation isn't the only wear and tear associated with aging. All too often, bones begin to thin out as we grow older because of a condition called osteoporosis. Chances are fair to good that you know someone with osteoporosis. Maybe you have it yourself. Up to 30 percent—nearly a third—of our bone can be lost to this condition.

Bone loss can begin as early as age 30, but it may go unnoticed until much later in life. Both men and women tend to lose bone mineral as they age. Five out of six osteoporosis victims, though, are women. Because women have a smaller bone mass to begin with—i.e., less bone to spare—they are more prone to the disabling effects of calcium loss. Strike one. For some reason, too, the drop-off in estrogen production that heralds menopause in women also accelerates bone loss. Srike two. A sudden fall—strike three—and the ball game's over. Each year, an estimated 100,000 women with bone loss suffered fractured hips (to say nothing of cracked vertebrae and broken arms). Half of them may die as an indirect result of their injuries, and the other half tend to lead very restricted lives—benched for the season, you might say.

Each of us—man or woman—can avoid that life-crippling problem, though. Part of the answer is exercise (see chapter 2), and the rest is paying special attention to calcium. After all, calcium is the primary mineral bones lose to osteoporosis.

Everett Smith, Ph.D., of the department of preventive medicine at the University of Wisconsin, is a specialist in aging and a pioneer in bone loss research. He told us, "The bone loss occurs from the bone marrow cavity—the center of the bone—while the outside structure, or bone diameter, remains the same size." That means the bone loses minerals—calcium and phosphorus—from the *inside*, and becomes more fragile. During the later years, a person's circulatory system also declines, and so fewer nutrients get to the cells, and some bone cells die.

Such cell death reduces a bone's ability to repair itself. With fewer living cells, the bone becomes more brittle. Stress on the bone can then cause tiny fatigue fractures; over time they may get larger and finally give way to a break.

The RDA for calcium is 800 milligrams a day. But it takes about 1,500 milligrams of calcium a day to stop or even reverse postmenopausal osteoporosis and the potentially fatal fractures blamed on it. Two cups of milk—still more than many adults are likely to drink daily—provide only 576 milligrams of calcium. The rest can be made up by eating yogurt, cheese and other dairy foods. But that means eating more dairy products than most people can add to their diet without stuffing themselves with calories and fat.

Fortunately, there are three bone-saving alternatives:

1. Exercise to help the body use the calcium it does get more efficiently (see chapter 2, Exercise Now).

2. Take bone meal or dolomite, both natural calcium products, to boost your calcium intake. (Bone meal is made from the powdered bones of animals; dolomite, from powdered rocks. Both are perfectly wholesome and edible.)

3. Better still, exercise *and* take calcium supplements. One doctor claims that bone loss between the ages of 30 and 70 can be reduced by as much as *half* with proper diet and exercise.

Dubious? Well, studies show that calcium supplements clearly help bones hold their own. Herta Spencer, M.D., and two colleagues at the Veterans Administration Hospital in Hines, Illinois, reported that an intake of 1,200 milligrams of calcium per day puts a halt to calcium's steady drain out of the bones (*NIH Record*, May 7, 1974). And a two-year study published in *Annals of Internal Medicine* (December, 1977) showed that 22 postmenopausal women who took 1,400 milligrams of calcium daily had *no* measurable bone loss.

And it's quite possible that calcium may even *reverse* bone loss! Calcium can add new density and strength to aging bones, according to a study conducted by a team of researchers led by Anthony A. Albanese, Ph.D., at the Miriam Osborn Memorial Home in Rye, New York, and the Burke Rehabilitation Center in nearby White Plains. Twelve elderly nursing home residents (all women) were each given 1,200 milligrams of calcium a day, in their diet and through supplements, plus vitamin D (essential for proper calcium utilization). Another group of women received no supplemental calcium. After three full years of boosted calcium, the women in the first group had denser bones. Even though they were now three years older, their bones were—for all practical purposes— actually younger! On the other hand, bone density in the women who had not received extra calcium continued to decrease. Dr. Albanese and his associates then tried giving calcium supplements to some younger postmenopausal women and women with fractures. After taking calcium supplements, both groups had stronger bones (*New York State Journal of Medicine,* February, 1975).

Vitamin D Helps Bones Use Calcium

Although calcium is the first consideration in building and keeping strong bones, our bodies cannot use calcium without vitamin D. The amount of vitamin D we get determines how much calcium is absorbed and how well it's used. When people do not get enough vitamin D, they may experience a different kind of bone fragility, a decrease in bone density that causes pain, tenderness and muscular weakness. This is called osteomalacia, or adult rickets.

Vitamin D is rarely found in foods. Our primary source of it is sunlight. Studies show that bones are weakest and most likely to break in winter and spring, when days are short, sunlight (and hence vitamin D) is scarce, and calcium stores in the body are low. Do you need to take vitamin D supplements? Maybe yes and maybe no. A study of 110 children in England produced evidence that in winter, vitamin D levels are determined more by summer exposure to the sun than by the foods we eat. Levels of vitamin D in the blood were higher in children who had been on vacation at the seashore the previous summer than in those who remained at home (*British Medical Journal,* January, 1979).

While basking at the seashore may be an excellent way to build up vitamin D in young people and middle-aged adults, older folks may have to rely on supplements the year 'round for theirs. In a study of 62 elderly patients, ranging in age from 65 to 95, sunlight appeared to have no effect on vitamin D levels in the blood. Those levels *did* increase, however, after the patients were given vitamin D supplements. The study concludes that older people may benefit more from taking vitamin D supplements than from regular doses of sunshine (*Gerontology,* vol. 24, 1978).

The RDA for vitamin D for older adults is 200 I.U. Because vitamin D is fat-soluble and therefore can be easily stored in the body, there's usually no need to exceed that amount.

Lecithin Tramples Cholesterol

Remember how exercise lowers cholesterol? Well, lecithin is a natural substance—available in supplement form—that can do the same thing. What the two provide is a double-barreled approach to fighting heart disease.

Lecithin has a long record in that fight. David Kritchevsky, Ph.D., a biochemist and associate director of the Wistar Institute of Anatomy and Biology in Philadelphia, told us that lecithin has been in the medical literature as a heart disease fighter for at least 30 years. A keen investigator of lecithin's powers, Dr. Kritchevsky told us, "We know that lecithin can actually reverse atherosclerosis in animals when it is *injected*. But people can't walk around with needle tracks on their arms. So we keep experimenting with lecithin given orally in people and in animals."

During the 1970s, studies in several countries cast a favorable light on the beneficial effects of lecithin—especially its ability to change the blood's proportion of high-density lipoproteins, or HDL (the good kind of cholesterol that seems to protect against atherosclerosis) to low-density lipoproteins, or LDL (the bad type that aids it). In general, the higher the proportion of HDL to LDL, the less chance there is of atherosclerosis and heart attack.

- Sweden, 1974: Five 50-year-old men took 1.7 grams of lecithin a day for nine weeks, while also abstaining from alcohol. Their HDL levels went up an average of 30 percent (*Nutrition and Metabolism*, vol. 17, no. 6, 1974).

- Australia, 1977: Three healthy people and seven patients with high cholesterol levels took 20 to 30 grams of lecithin per day for periods ranging from eight weeks to 11 months. In one of the healthy persons and in three of the seven patients there was a significant drop in cholesterol. Furthermore, when lecithin was combined with clofibrate—a cholesterol-lowering drug— cholesterol levels fell even further (an average of 21.5 percent). Finally, that fall in cholesterol levels was "almost totally accounted for by a reduction in LDL" (*Australian and New Zealand Journal of Medicine*, June, 1977).

- Italy, 1978: Twenty-one people with elevated cholesterol levels took 1.8 grams of lecithin per day, drank no alcohol, and cut down on their intake of saturated fats. The cholesterol of more than 92 percent of the people with elevated LDL returned to normal levels. "The present results," said the researchers, "underline the therapeutic value of [lecithin] in hyperlipemic patients [those with elevated cholesterol]" (*Current Therapeutic Research*, August, 1978).

And now in the 1980s, there is every indication that lecithin studies will continue to tell good tales. At Rutgers Medical School, for example, researchers are studying the effects of a specially formulated all-polyunsaturated lecithin. Twelve people who had elevated cholesterol and coronary artery disease took 30 grams of the lecithin daily for 16 weeks. While not affecting the cholesterol levels themselves, the lecithin raised an important HDL factor, prompting the researchers to conclude that lecithin may exert "a favorable effect" against atherosclerosis (*American Journal of Clinical Nutrition*, April, 1980).

Lecithin Works Best with a Low-Fat Diet

Ronald K. Tompkins, M.D., of the department of surgery, University of California at Los Angeles School of Medicine, has recently reported on his study of four men and one woman, 64 to 84 years of age, who took 48 grams of lecithin a day for 24 months. They also reduced their fat intake to 50 grams per day and dropped their cholesterol levels to 300 milligrams by cutting out fried foods and saturated fats. "The entire group showed a decrease in cholesterol values during the low-fat and lecithin combinations," said Dr. Tompkins. Indeed, the average drop in cholesterol was 22 percent (*American Journal of Surgery*, vol. 140, no. 3, 1980). "At this point we're not certain," Dr. Tompkins told us "but we think that it may be important to combine lecithin with a low-fat diet to really do the trick."

Lecithin occurs naturally in human, animal and vegetable cells. As a supplement, soybean lecithin is sold as a liquid, in liquid-filled capsules, and in granular form. The granular form is the most concentrated—one tablespoon equals approximately ten 1,200-milligram capsules. Granulated lecithin can be taken as is, sprinkled in soups or salads, added to gravies, sauces and dressings or mixed in juice or milk.

The effects of lecithin vary from person to person. With some, it has a dramatic effect, raising HDL and lowering LDL levels or lowering total cholesterol. With others, the effects are minimal. But the same can be said of drugs (like clofibrate) that are taken to lower cholesterol and that, moreover, can have serious side effects.

Keep in mind, too, that when lecithin is not as effective as hoped in changing cholesterol levels, exercise can make up the difference. (See chapter 2 for more details on exercise.)

So whether you're after bones that last a lifetime, cells that resist years of wear and tear, or arteries that stay cholesterol free, superior nutrition is plainly the first place to look.

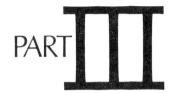

PART **III**

A Personal Road Map for Long Life

Antidotes to Stress

CHAPTER 7

Think of stress and you probably think of things like office politics, financial pressure, illness in the family or a disagreement with your spouse. Throw in a broken shoelace or lost car keys and composure can crumble like a sand castle at high tide. You don't need a book to tell you that all kinds of hassles—big or small—produce anxiety. But did you know that stress and anxiety can shorten your life?

Well, they can. The reason is that stress produces adrenaline, a hormone so potent it can flood the body with superhuman strength. You've undoubtedly heard of instances in which a panic-stricken individual lifted a two-ton car to free a child pinned under the wheels. The stimulant was adrenaline. Secreted by the adrenal glands during periods of stress, adrenaline (also called "epinephrine" by scientists) electrifies the system for quick action. The heart races. The liver releases stored blood sugar (glucose), and blood pressure shoots up, forcing that sugar to the muscles and brain. The pupils dilate. The intestines shut down. Breathing is short and rapid. You feel tense, apprehensive, ready.

If there's a two-ton car to be moved, fine. All that pent-up anxiety can be put to good use. But should the rush of adrenaline spring from a less than do-or-die situation—a traffic jam or other hassle of daily life—your body doesn't really need it, and you stew in your own juice. When you secrete adrenaline on a daily basis, maybe an *hourly* basis, you weaken your heart, your blood vessels, your entire body. Here's the proof.

■ People with high blood pressure have higher levels of adrenaline circulating in their blood than people with normal blood pressure (*Journal of Clinical Pharmacology*, September, 1979).

■ In 52 people who suffered a heart attack, the average excretion of adrenaline among the 9 who died was much higher than among the 43 who survived (*Nature*, May 3, 1969).

■ In 1979 researchers at Yale University School of Medicine found that adrenaline "negatively affects" glucose metabolism—the way the body handles blood sugar. "Someone under stress secretes an increased amount of epinephrine," David Diebert, M.D., one of the researchers, told us. "And with that increase the liver secretes too much glucose and the tissues absorb too little."

To sum up: "One is compelled to believe that the adrenaline continually released during chronic stress has negative physical effects," said Jonathan Moss, M.D., Ph.D., a researcher from Harvard Medical School who has studied adrenaline.

Big and Little Hassles
Add Up to Stress

It's not necessarily the size of a hassle, but how it affects our day-to-day life that makes the difference in whether or not our adrenaline launches deadly hit-and-run assaults. Take a man who learns that his brother, who lived in another state, has suddenly died. He'll grieve at the loss, but chances are that after the funeral his life will go on with little or no change. Should his business partner die, however, the man would not only feel the personal loss of a friend but would probably also have to deal with a host of small hassles in carrying on without his partner. The second incident would be more stressful than the first.

Similarly, the death of a spouse can be less stressful than life with an alcoholic mate. Getting fired can be less stressful than working for a tactless, overbearing boss. Sending your firstborn off to college can be less stressful than living under the same roof with a temperamental teenager. What's more, you're under constant pressure, petty problems that might be ignored—a cluttered room or cranky child—can rub you the wrong way, unleashing a fresh surge of adrenaline.

Some people automatically react to stress—routine or cataclysmic—by distracting themselves by watching more TV, drinking too much, taking tranquilizers, or sleeping more. That's not coping—it's taking the path of least resistance. Sooner or later, troubles have to be dealt with, for life is inherently stressful in one way or another. The real way to prevent the lethal effects of stress and its assault of adrenaline is to learn to, first, spare yourself unnecessary stress, and second, deal appropriately with unavoidable troubles.

Nine Stress Reducers
That Can Save Your Life

1. CUT THE COFFEE. Ever find yourself feeling tense and jumpy when there's nothing to be tense about? That could be due to any one of a number of bad habits that manufacture extra adrenaline. Drinking coffee, for instance. Caffeine in coffee (and tea, chocolate and cola drinks) makes many people feel jittery and tense. Scientists strongly suspect that caffeine stimulates the adrenal glands to pump out the hormone. In one study, the average adrenaline level of non-coffee drinkers more than tripled after they drank a cup of coffee—a level as high as that of someone given nitroglycerin, a powerful stimulant (*New England Journal of Medicine*, January, 1978).

In its discussion of caffeine, the American Pharmaceutical Association *Handbook of Nonprescription Drugs* (5th edition, 1979) says, "Doses larger than 250 milligrams often cause insomnia, restlessness, irritability, nervousness, tremor, headaches, and, in rare instances, a mild form of delirium manifested as perceived noises and flashes of light"—symptoms almost identical to classic signs of anxiety.

How much coffee must you drink to reach the danger point of 250 milligrams? The average cup of coffee will deliver about 100 milligrams of caffeine, so it takes only 2½ cups to make you a candidate for restlessness and all the rest. (A cup of tea has from 50 to 100 milligrams of caffeine, depending on its strength.) It takes anywhere from 30 minutes to two hours for caffeine to spark the release of adrenaline, and another three to ten hours for your body to rid itself of just half the caffeine you've consumed. Conceivably, then, even just two or three well-spaced cups of coffee or tea every day could put you on a round-the-clock caffeine high. And that unrelenting barrage of adrenaline is very stressful to your whole body.

2. NIX NICOTINE. Cigarettes are no kinder to your adrenaline system than coffee. A study shows that adrenaline levels are 20 percent higher on a day when a person smokes than on a day when he doesn't (*Journal of Clinical Pharamacology*, July, 1977). No wonder a novice smoker becomes nauseated, pale and sweaty when he lights up.

3. NO NIGHTCAPS. Alcohol, too, riles up the adrenal glands—

especially if you also smoke cigarettes and drink coffee. Says Herbert Sprince, Ph.D., a researcher at the Veterans Administration Hospital in Coatesville, Pennsylvania, "There is a considerable body of evidence that the intake of alcohol, the smoking of cigarettes and the drinking of coffee release catecholamines." (Adrenaline is one of a group of hormones that scientists label catecholamines.)

4. EXERCISE. Some people *like* the rush of adrenaline that follows a cup of coffee or a cigarette, and they don't want anything to bring them down. In fact, they may be so addicted to adrenaline that they not only gorge on stimulants but also purposely put themselves in stressful situations that give them a rise. And perhaps that's understandable. Adrenaline is a natural stimulant, and one that our bodies seem to relish. The problem with stimulants—and stress-induced adrenaline—however, is that too much is released too fast.

What you really need is a harmless way to get a moderate jolt of adrenaline, a way to feel invigorated and alert that doesn't sizzle your health. What you need instead of coffee, cigarettes and contrived hassles is *exercise*, which gives your body an adrenaline lift without dropping you flat on your face. The facts speak for themselves.

Minutes after nine men had exercised, scientists measured their adrenaline levels and found the average level was 50 percent higher than before exercise (*Journal of the American Medical Association*, January 25, 1980). In a similar experiment, the average epinephrine level of over 50 people more than doubled after exercise (*Journal of Clinical Pharmacology*, September, 1979).

The advantage of exercise-induced adrenaline output is that exercise puts the adrenaline to work. Running, playing racquetball or taking a brisk stroll burns up the stimulant so that it doesn't burn you out. Exercise delivers adrenaline as nature intended it to be delivered—healthfully.

*   *   *   *   *

Even without coffee, cigarettes or manufactured crises, life has its stresses. Here are some tips on disarming those troubles.

5. TALK IT OUT. Ernest Harburg, Ph.D., told us that discussing problems that cause angry feelings may release them harmlessly or may even prevent them from welling up in the first place.

"The discuss approach," Dr. Harburg said, "which we are just beginning to understand, is a way in which you explore the problem in a detached manner. You acknowledge your anger, but you are not openly hostile, verbally or physically. Discussion involves detachment, reflection, conversation and a willingness to solve the problem." Dr. Harburg feels that the discuss approach works because it removes the cause of anger.

Dr. Harburg's conclusions are based on work done at the University of Michigan School of Public Health, where he and other researchers studied the blood pressures of people who became angry when unfairly confronted by authority figures. "Those who bottle up their anger have the highest blood pressures, and those who became openly hostile have the second highest blood pressures. People who take action to resolve their anger have the lowest pressures," the researchers noted (*University of Michigan News*, June 25, 1980).

A classic study, begun in 1946 among students at the Johns Hopkins University School of Medicine, compared psychological tests administered while the students were in school with their health records in later years. People who got cancer tended to prefer being alone when stressed rather than confiding in others or seeking advice. Interestingly, that tendency to withdraw was also shared by people who committed suicide (*Johns Hopkins Medical Journal*, October, 1980).

6. HAVE A GOOD CRY. Many psychiatrists and psychologists also believe that crying relieves stress.

"Crying discharges tension, the accumulation of feeling associated with whatever problem is causing the crying," said Frederic Flach, M.D., associate clinical professor in psychiatry at Cornell University Medical College in New York City, and author of *Choices* (Bantam, 1979). And since crying is a healthy, natural form of communication, learning *not* to cry makes us unhealthy—and, in terms of human development, less fit to survive.

"Emotions developed over the course of evolution as a way to communicate, a way for a person to have his intentions understood and to insure his survival," said research psychologist Robert Plutchik, Ph.D., professor of psychiatry and psychology at Albert Einstein College of Medicine, and author of *Emotion: A Psychoevolutionary Synthesis* (Harper & Row, 1979). "The suppression of crying, which is often learned in this society, leads the individual to inhibit all the other emotions he feels when he is hurt, such as fear, anxiety and anger. This inhibits the individual's effectiveness and decreases the likelihood that humans will survive. It's very important to communicate feelings during times of stress."

7. QUIT WORRYING. As we said earlier, how we react to problems determines the amount of stress we then feel. All too often, we react to existing or potential problems by worrying about them. Some of our worries are painfully real, others are the by-products of a feverish imagination. Either way, worrying can stir up adrenaline.

"Most worries are anticipatory worries," said Barry Lubetkin, Ph.D., a psychologist at the Institute for Behavior Therapy in New York City. "We're afraid of what *might* happen."

Even still, worries aren't a big stress until they begin to dominate your everyday life. Dr. Lubetkin explained several techniques he uses to help anxious and worried people.

One is called *coping desensitization*. If you're worried about a problem in the future—financial trouble or a conflict with someone, for example—imagine yourself in the fearful situation. Then imagine that you are coping with it, or even enjoying it. A person who fears airplanes might replace his or her terror with positive images, such as the view from the window or a pleasant chat with a new acquaintance.

Another technique is called *cognitive tracking*, or *reality testing*. Ask yourself if your worries are supported by the facts. In similar situations in the past, were you unable to cope? A man afraid of failing to sexually satisfy his wife should ask himself if he failed before. If not, he can stop worrying. That method works if you set aside 15 or 20 minutes a day to relax and think the problem through, said Dr. Lubetkin.

Then there's the *worst case* method. If the future looks bleak, try imagining the worst possible outcomes. For an accident at home, imagine cuts, poisoning, broken bones. For a long auto trip, imagine flat tires and running out of gas. Ask yourself if the worst would really be all that bad, and imagine yourself coping with it.

Sometimes we just can't put our finger on what's bothering us, though. For someone who suffers from nameless dread, Dr. Lubetkin suggests *time sampling*. In that method, the worrier devotes the last ten minutes of every hour to writing down in a journal the things his or her mind is dwelling on. That helps isolate and identify the "themes of worry," said Dr. Lubetkin.

There are certain kinds of worries that we bring home with us from work. It would be better to leave our problems—like our muddy boots—outside the door. One man designated a tree by his house as his "worry tree," Dr. Lubetkin told us. Every day after work he "hung" his worries on a branch of the worry tree, and left them there until morning. It was a ritual that worked for him, and one psychiatrist, Herbert C. Modlin, M.D., calls such rituals "absolutely legitimate" for coping with worry.

As a senior psychiatrist at the Menninger Foundation in

Topeka, Kansas, Dr. Modlin has seen several ways professionals and executives insulate their home lives from the tensions of the workday. One man sets aside the hour from 6 to 7 P.M. for playing with his two young sons. They play catch or basketball in season, or work on stamp collections or Cub Scout projects together. That ritual pays off double dividends: the man sheds his tensions and relieves his worry that he might be neglecting his children.

"Anything that shifts our concentration to something else, that provides a change of pace, is a legitimate device," said Dr. Modlin. "A change of mental content, such as meditation or yoga, will work, too."

8. TAKE RELAXATION BREAKS. Speaking of meditation, one way to break the momentum of galloping anxiety—worry-induced or otherwise—is to put all systems temporarily on hold. Whether you're at home or in the office, close the door, take the phone off the hook, shut your eyes and *do nothing* for 10 or 15 minutes. Better yet, take a few deep breaths and concentrate on a pleasant image. Or do a few slow stretches. Whatever you decide to try, do it twice a day. The rewards in terms of well-being are larger than you might imagine. R. Keith Wallace, Ph.D., chairman of the biology department at Maharishi International University in Fairfield, Iowa, reports that Transcendental Meditation (TM), a stress-control technique that produces a tranquil state of mind, actually slows aging. "We've found that the longer a person practices TM, the greater the decrease in biological age," said Dr. Wallace.

9. LEARN TO SAY MAÑANA. That means "tomorrow" in Spanish. In a larger sense, it also means "no rush," as anyone who's traveled in a Spanish-speaking country can tell you. But rather than get impatient at the more relaxed pace of life there, we'd all be better off adopting it for ourselves.

Something called Type A behavior made a lot of headlines a couple of years ago when it was found that a time-urgent personality seems to predict coronary disease and heart attacks. People who are hard-driving, achievement-oriented, time-conscious, competitive and hostile, it seems, are not likely to be rewarded with a long life. Type B's, on the other hand, tend to get just as much done, but without killing themselves in the process.

Are you a Type A? You might be, if you:
- Try to do two things at once—like reading while you drive or walk the dog.
- Can't stand to wait in line.
- Gesticulate while you talk.

- Speak explosively.
- Finish other people's sentences.
- Nod your head or click your lips while listening.
- Have a fetish about always being on time.
- Play every game to win.
- Believe that if you want something done right, you have to do it yourself.
- Measure success in terms of numbers—number of memos written, clients seen, and so on.

If you fit that description, don't panic. Because time urgency is the underlying trait of Type A behavior, the best way to beat it is to take time less seriously. You needn't do everything by your watch. Learn to say *mañana*.

Adopt that and as many of the other stress antidotes as you can and you'll be pleasantly surprised at how unburdened you begin to feel. And you'll probably live longer for it. Robert Samp, M.D., of the University of Wisconsin Medical School faculty, studied 7,000 people, young and old, and learned some fascinating things about mental attitude and longevity.

"The greater emphasis we found in older people was on a certain inner peace," Dr. Samp explained. Sometimes that meant an adjustment in lifestyle. "The inactive became more involved," said Dr. Samp, "and the folks burning the candle at both ends began burning it at only one end instead."

Dr. Samp's observations support other psychologists who say that people who live a long life have developed an ability to cope. "People who are dynamic, impetuous, driving and uptight [classic Type A behavior] are not displaying qualities that will help them reach old age," said Dr. Samp. On the other hand, "the long-lived people aren't killing themselves from the inside out. During their sojourn through life, they have learned to pace themselves."

Follow the antistress advice in this chapter and you might achieve that perfect pace—and an enjoyable stroll to a longer life.

Smoking and Drinking, Shortcuts to Old Age

CHAPTER 8

The time was when smoking, drinking and carrying on were about the worst things a lady could do to her good name. Well, society may have grown more tolerant, but our bodies—both men's and women's—haven't; they still can't abide these habits without serious protest—and damage.

Thank You for Not Smoking

When actor Humphrey Bogart found out he had cancer of the esophagus (food pipe) in 1956, he continued to smoke because, as he said, "your esophagus has nothing to do with your lungs."

Sorry, Bogie, but you were wrong on that. Lung cancer is not the only cancer associated with cigarettes. Cancers of the throat, mouth and the esophagus are also linked to smoking, especially when alcohol is involved. (Bogie, of course, was known to indulge in more than an occasional drink.)

In 1978, lung cancer and other respiratory cancers killed 99,000 people, which was one-fourth of all the deaths due to cancer in the United States. Cigarettes probably accounted for 80 to 85 percent of those deaths, according to the *Journal of the National Cancer Institute* (December, 1979). But smoking affects other vital organs as well:

- Smoking just one cigarette a day increases the risk of gastric cancer.
- Smokers have higher rates of pancreatic and bladder cancer than nonsmokers.

■ Men who smoke are more likely to develop kidney cancer than men who don't smoke.
■ Women who smoke are more prone to cervical cancer than women who don't smoke.

And, if by some miracle all those organs escape the fatal effects of the weed, a smoker is still not home free. His or her heart may knuckle under. Cigarette smoking is one of the most common causes of fatal heart attacks, according to the *Journal of the American Medical Association* (May 15, 1981). Along the same lines, smoking also speeds up the hardening of the arteries (arteriosclerosis) and causes increases in blood pressure.

Put those gruesome facts all together, and it's possible to say that a smoker doubles his or her chances of dying by the age of 65. No wonder a leading aging specialist referred to smoking as "sucking on death."

Smoking Hastens Aging

Not only do smokers die sooner than they ought to, but the effects of smoking often mimic effects of "old age," and smoking may even *speed* aging:

MEMORY IS SMOKED OUT. Before you get annoyed at someone for forgetting your name, note whether he or she smokes. According to a study by a Scottish psychologist, chronic cigarette smokers are more likely to forget people's names than nonsmokers. Dr. David J. Weeks, citing the U.S. Surgeon General's report on smoking and health, suggests that the poor memories of smokers are due to generalized atherosclerosis. Smoking may impair blood supply to the brain and leave smokers groping for names (*British Medical Journal*, December 22–29, 1979).

If someone you know frequently returns from the store with only half the items he or she set out to buy, smoking could again be the cause. Researchers at the University of California at Los Angeles tested the memory of smokers by asking them to recall items from a 75-item list after some smoked regular cigarettes and others tried nicotine-free cigarettes. In each case, recall was tested immediately after smoking and again two days later. Both immediate and delayed recall of the items was considerably poorer when people smoked cigarettes containing nicotine (*American Journal of Psychiatry*, February, 1978).

A FASTER TRIP TO MENOPAUSE. Women who are wont to light up are apt to roll down the road to menopause at an earlier age than their nonsmoking sisters. So said three Boston researchers who reviewed the case histories of more than 3,500 middle-aged women in seven countries. After categorizing the women according to their age, menopausal status and smoking habits, the researchers discovered that in each age group there were invariably more smokers past menopause than nonsmokers. By age 51, for example, 79 percent of those who smoked more than a pack a day had already undergone menopause, compared to only 56 percent of those who never took a puff. Furthermore, the study suggested that the more cigarettes a woman smokes each day, the earlier her menopause is likely to occur (*Lancet*, June 25, 1977).

We could go on and on. A list of smoking's ill effects would be almost endless and would include a crippled circulatory system, infertility in men, shortness of breath, a hacking cough and premature wrinkles, to name just a few. (To say nothing of bad breath!)

It's Never Too Late to Quit

If you're hooked on cigarettes, don't avoid quitting simply because you think the damage to your health has already been done. Dr. J. H. Abramson, from the Hebrew University-Hadassah Medical School, Jerusalem, Israel, investigated some statistics on longevity and smoking and found that men who gave up smoking as late as their sixties and seventies still lived longer than men of that age who continued to smoke. Specifically, Dr. Abramson found that men between the ages of 65 and 74 who continued to smoke had a 24 percent higher death rate than those who quit. For smokers aged 75 to 84, the death rate remained 12 percent higher than for quitters (*American Journal of the Medical Sciences*, July/August, 1977).

To help you quit—no matter how old you are—many churches and YMCAs have smoking liberation classes. Commercial no-smoking classes are usually listed in the Yellow Pages of the phone directory under "Smokers Information and Treatment Centers."

Alcohol's Effects Also Mimic Old Age and Shorten Life

Any college student knows that alcohol kills brain cells. And those cells don't revive—ever. Medically, that's called "cerebral atrophy." But because we've each got around 100 billion brain cells to work with, most people assume that they can spare a few without worrying. To a degree, they're right. Still, what no one seems to know is just how many brain cells we can lose without seriously, permanently compromising brain function. True, it's a matter of individual susceptibility. Yet brain cells are a precious commodity, and the fact remains that the more alcohol we drink, the more we risk draining our brains.

One of the problems this drain causes is that an alcohol-beleaguered brain has trouble remembering things. Things like where its owner parked the car...or put the keys. A drinker's brain also learns things more slowly and has trouble with complicated concepts. In fact, the lapses of memory, confusion and slowed reflexes produced by a lifetime of steady, heavy tippling closely resemble the doddering traits of senility that we hope to dodge in old age. That this is true should not be all that surprising, because both cerebral atrophy and senility are physically rooted in some form of brain damage. So why court somthing that amounts to pseudosenility?

But besides making us act old before our time, drinking—like smoking—can actually shorten life.

From time to time we hear medical reports that claim that moderate drinkers (people who average two drinks a day) are less likely to have heart attacks than either heavy drinkers or teetotalers. That moderate drinkers are better off than heavy drinkers we don't question. After all, alcoholics aren't generally known for their longevity. But abstainers? Can a couple of nips a night actually contribute to long life?

Not really. The theory is that a couple of beers, two glasses of wine, or a double highball raises blood levels of HDL (high-density lipoproteins), a constituent of cholesterol believed to protect against heart disease. The catch here is that even though moderate drinkers may suffer fewer heart attacks, one study shows they do not necessarily live longer than either their teetotaling or besotted neighbors. Moderate drinkers simply die from causes other than heart disease—causes often aggravated by alcohol. In fact, another study concluded that habitual imbibing may offset the benefit of increased HDL by upping the risk of accidents, stroke and cancer (*Canadian Medical Association Journal*, November 22, 1980).

Less Drinking Means Fewer Accidents

We probably can't tell you much about drinking and car accidents that you don't already know. Drinking drivers frequently crack up because when alcohol reaches the brain, their field of vision narrows. And even after only moderate drinking, they experience temporary but critical difficulties in noticing objects—like stop signs, oncoming cars or pedestrians. Four drinks consumed in three hours (the amount the average drinker might have at a party or a ball game) supply more than enough alcohol to seriously impair driving skills. Braking and steering ability become erratic then, and critical, split-second decisions are delayed—or made poorly. And, of course, drunken pedestrians experience the same difficulties and dangers negotiating busy intersections.

What's more, accidental traffic deaths aren't the only alcohol-related tragedies. The same cloudy reasoning and poor coordination can contribute to fatal fires. A U.S. government survey states that 83 percent of the middle-aged men who die in fires are drinking before or at the time of the accident.

Raise a Glass
and Raise Your Blood Pressure

Even if we don't drive while drinking, we could be on the road to trouble. Alcohol can also send blood pressure soaring, increasing our chances for stroke. Researchers at the University of Tasmania (located off the southern coast of Australia) completed a study that suggests "any alcohol consumption is associated with increased blood pressure." The researchers interviewed 85 physically active men to find out their age, height, weight, smoking habits, salt consumption, alcohol intake and family history. They also took the men's blood pressures. Finally, they analyzed all the information they had collected. Of all the variables considered, alcohol consumption appeared to be the main contributor to high blood pressure. Further, the researchers concluded that up to 10 percent of all high blood pressure could be blamed on drinking alcohol (*Medical Journal of Australia*, August 23, 1980).

Such evidence suggests that people with high blood pressure not drink at all. And for good reason. Heavy alcohol consumption has also been linked to stroke, a common upshot of high blood pressure. A study of the case histories of 76 people at the University of Helsinki, Finland, for example, found that even occasional intoxication seems to increase the risk of stroke in young adults. Scientists at the department of neurology there noticed that in a random examination of their heart cases, strokes in young patients were often preceded by drinking bouts. A look at the medical records for all stroke patients under the age of 40 revealed a definite pattern—when drinking went up, the possibility of stroke did too. Fifteen of the 76 people were stricken within 24 hours of a drinking spree, and 2 suffered strokes while still drunk. Over half the cases were reported on weekends when drinking in Finland is heaviest (*Lancet*, December 2, 1978).

Smoking and Drinking,
a Cancer Double-Whammy

When it comes to cancer, smoking is bad, but smoking *and* drinking is worse. Not surprisingly, the head and neck areas— mouth, tongue, throat, esophagus and larynx (voice box) seem to be the most sensitive to alcohol-induced cancer. Those tissues are flooded with alcohol and irritated by smoking residues. When any two carcinogens (cancer-causing substances) go to work on the same vulnerable tissues (as they do in this case), cancer cells tend to materialize more readily and quickly than they would without either the alcohol or the cigarettes.

In addition to alcohol's direct link to cancer, drinking weakens parts of our immune system that are already fading with advancing age. Alcohol robs the body of vitamins and minerals that we need to stay healthy and resistant to disease. And alcohol reduces the number of lymphocytes in the blood; these cells help the immune system fight off not only carcinogens but viruses and bacteria as well.

Add all the direct drawbacks of smoking and drinking—various cancers, heart disease, stroke and untold respiratory distress—to their indirect devilments—such as loss of memory, fuzzy mental capacity, poor motor ability, loss of friends and reduced life span. Try as we might, then, we just can't find anything good to say about smoking or drinking. (Incidentally, low-tar and low-nicotine brands are not "health sticks." People who smoke them still tend to die sooner than nonsmokers.) We don't know where the ad people find all their praises for the comforts of smoking and the pleasures of relaxing with a drink, but we'll let them worry about it. It's a matter of conscience, we guess. We'll just leave it at the suggestion that you give up both.

Accidents Don't Have to Happen

CHAPTER 9

Accidents are the fourth biggest cause of death in America. Only heart disease, cancer and stroke kill more people than accidents do. So avoiding accidents—at home, on the highway, or at work—is just as important to living a long life as eating the right foods or not smoking.

We actually have more control over accidents than we think we do. Of course, some mishaps are simply a matter of bad luck. But most of us also go through occasional periods of klutziness, for which there are perfectly good explanations. Often, we become easy marks merely because we're under stress and out of shape.

Stress Breeds Blunders

"During stressful periods in life, your odds of having an accident increase," concluded Abraham Bergman, M.D., a researcher at the University of Washington in Seattle, after conducting a study of 103 junior high school boys. For five months the boys reported both accidents and "life changes" (such as moving to a new school or an illness in the family) to the doctor. After the reports were in, Dr. Bergman and two colleagues compared the list of life changes with the number of accidents. The boys under little stress from change had a total of 395 accidents; the boys under lots of stress had 946 (*Pediatrics*, August, 1976). Clearly, stress bred accident-proneness.

In a similar study, two researchers from the University of Michigan asked over 500 men for information on the stress in their lives over the past year and the number of car accidents they had had. Then the researchers placed the stresses next to the accidents to see if they matched up. They did. Stress bred accident-proneness again.

Life changes and stress "are significantly related to traffic accidents," the researchers wrote. The events most likely to "predict" accidents were "physical stress responses" such as smoking, insomnia, headaches and ulcers; problems with parents or in-laws; problems or pressure in school or on the job; or financial troubles (*American Journal of Psychiatry*, August, 1974).

Why does stress foster mishaps? And what can you do about it?

"People who are under a lot of stress are likely candidates for accidents—big and small—because they can't think, act or react in a normal, relaxed manner," said William Simons, supervisor of safety management programs for Pennsylvania State University's Institute of Public Safety. Instead of having his attention on the task at hand, the stressed person is preoccupied, Simons told us.

"Stress is very significant, because should a person be having problems, at home, with his marriage, his children, his finances or whatever, he definitely won't be able to pay 100 percent attention to what he's doing," said Simons. "When the individual is preoccupied with problems, when he or she is tense and worried, that's when accidents often occur."

Another way that stress sets you up for an accident is by wearing down your energy reserves. Fatigue is a reaction to stress, says a report in the *New York State Journal of Medicine* (July, 1980).

And even when fatigue comes from the wear and tear of a typical day and not from stress, it still lays you wide open for a mishap. "Law enforcement officers have statistics to prove that casualties increase as the day grows older," said a report in *California Highway Patrolman* (December, 1967). "The climax is reached in the late afternoon and evening hours. Drivers are tired. Their reflexes are dull."

What to do about stress? Above all, don't reach for tranquilizers. A British study showed that drivers who use Valium or other so-called minor tranquilizers are five times more likely to have a car accident than people not taking a tranquilizer (*British Medical Journal*, April 7, 1979).

A better idea is to deal with stress directly—be aware that you are under stress and becoming more accident-prone. "A sure sign of increasing stress is a series of minor accidents," said Simons, who advises people to "be on guard" if they begin having too many minor mishaps. That's a must, he warned, because "increased frequency will soon lead to increased severity."

Next, give yourself a change of pace. One study that compared a high-accident group of people to a low-accident group found that the low-accident folks took more vacations. And a psychiatrist investigating people who had suffered disabling accidents found that during the year before their accident they had experienced fewer "socially desirable events"—that there had been too few pleasant surprises in their lives. A break in your routine could avert a break in your leg, it seems.

Fitness Is No Accident

People might be less tired and thus sharper in the late afternoon, and so less likely to have an accident, if they were more fit. People who exercise regularly don't tire as easily as folks who don't, and they don't fall victim to accidents as easily, either. "The degree of fitness many times determines whether there will be an accident or whether one will be avoided," said Charles Peter Yost, Ph.D., professor and dean emeritus at West Virginia University. Dr. Yost told us that fitness prevents accidents by contributing to both our mental sharpness and our physical readiness to stop an accident before it starts. Being fit means being strong enough to regain one's footing after stumbling on the stairs or slipping on a newly waxed floor.

"In skiing, for example, the most important single prevention of ski injury lies in proper conditioning," said Dr. Yost. He also described his study of a skiing school in Lake Placid, New York. The first year he watched the school's 50 children, they had a total of seven fractures and five sprains among them after 5,000 hours of skiing. The next year's class, however, had no accidents though they skied as much, thanks to a preclass conditioning program (*National Safety Congress Transactions*, vol. 23, 1966).

Diets and Downfalls

Weight, too, can be a risk factor. The more pounds we rack up on the scale, the more we are apt to fumble and tumble.

"Significantly overweight people—those who are more than 30 percent above their ideal weight—have an increase in accident-proneness," said Willard Krehl, M.D., professor emeritus of Jefferson Medical College in Philadelphia. And, Dr. Krehl added, "the tendency toward accidents increases as the person gets heavier." To make matters worse, overweight people may become even more accident-prone if they take diet pills—or other medications that fog the brain.

Skipping breakfast—to lose weight or save time—can also

contribute to accidents. Researchers in England found that the number of accidents on the job among forge workers decreased if the laborers—who usually ate very little breakfast—had more under their belts in the morning. The researchers divided the workers into three groups. At midmorning, one group received a high-energy drink, rich in carbohydrate. A second group received the same quantity of liquid, but their drink was much lower in carbohydrate. A third group didn't get anything. After four months, the researchers tabulated the number of accidents in the three groups. The result: the men who received the high-carbohydrate drink had the fewest accidents, and the men who got nothing had the most. The researchers said that the carbohydrate-deprived workers were suffering from something called "transient malnutrition"; it caused fatigue, and that led to the accidents (*Scandinavian Journal of Work Environment and Health*, January, 1980).

As simple as it sounds, regular meals, regular exercise and regular breaks from both work *and* routine go a long way toward foiling personal calamities.

Live It Up

CHAPTER 10

So far, we've discussed many ways to help outrun the physical aspects of aging. But there's more to longevity than top physical health. While the human body has the capacity to last up to 120 years, the stress of life can make us ready to quit long before then—unless, of course, we learn to weather stress and face life with a healthful attitude. In many ways, a long, full life is a matter of choice.

People Need People

In 1974 Harold and Bertha Soderquist joined the Peace Corps. He was 80 and she was 76. Although the Peace Corps does not expect its volunteers past 50 to do well in language training, the Soderquists went out and passed with honors. The oldest volunteers ever in the Peace Corps, the Soderquists then were sent to Western Samoa to teach secondary school.

The Soderquists were people involved with people, and that connection may be a significant factor in increasing longevity. That's the conclusion, at least, of a study of Alameda County, California, in which Lisa F. Berkman, Ph.D., of Yale University, and S. Leonard Syme, Ph.D., of the University of California at Berkeley, evaluated the effects of social and community ties on longevity. Sources of social contact were defined as marriage, close friendships and family ties, church affiliations, and other informal and formal group associations.

The study showed that men who were most isolated from others had a mortality rate 2.3 times greater than men with the most social connections, while women had a mortality rate that was 2.8 times higher. The figures also show that the more isolated a person is, the more likely that person is to die of heart disease, circulatory diseases, cancer, digestive- and respiratory-system diseases, and even accidents (*American Journal of Epidemiology*, February, 1979).

At a symposium of scientists called "The Healing Brain," held in New York City in December, 1980, Dr. Berkman elaborated on her findings. For example, she pointed out that she had found one important psychological factor that could also predict good health: how satisfied people were with their lives in general. Thus, if you have a good social life, and you also feel good about your life, you may be even healthier.

Dr. Berkman also noted that no matter how good your health practices are, if you are socially isolated they may not do you much good. "Social ties predicted mortality independently of cigarette smoking, alcohol consumption, obesity, sleeping and eating patterns, and utilization of preventive health services," said Dr. Berkman.

Scientists are quick to admit that they do not know exactly why people who have a lot of social contact live longer than those who don't. All sorts of reasons have been proposed: people may tell other people about good health practices, or sociable people may feel less depressed, or social contact may help the immune system ward off diseases.

In any case, Dr. Berkman feels that "loving and nurturing may be as important as *being* loved and nurtured." Such an idea is supported by George E. Vaillant, M.D., in his book *Adaptation to Life* (Little, Brown, 1977).

Dr. Vaillant is the current director of the Grant Study, which since 1939 has been following various aspects of the lives and careers of a group of Harvard University graduates. Of the men that Dr. Vaillant has worked with, he has been able to categorize 40 as either "friendly" or "lonely"—that is, those who have the capacity to love and those who do not.

Of all the ways he has subdivided the men of the Grant Study, Dr. Vaillant said that his categories of friendly and lonely have "proved the most dramatic." Among other things, the capacity to love was associated with "subsequent physical and mental health. Half of the lonely but only one of the friendly had developed a chronic physical illness by age 52. At some point in their adult lives, half of the lonely but only two of the friendly could have been called mentally ill."

Writing in the *American Journal of Medicine* (April, 1979), Leon Eisenberg, M.D., has perhaps summed up the people-who-need-people situation most eloquently. "There are, of course, no pharmacies available to fill a prescription for 'spouses, confidants and friends, p.r.n. [as needed]'," said Dr. Eisenberg, but "the point remains that social isolation is in itself a pathogenic factor in disease production. Mechanisms of social bonding are as ancient as the evolution of our species; their disruption has devastating impact. Good friends are an essential ingredient for good health."

Optimists Live Longer

"Loneliness is a terrible enemy," said Robert Samp, M.D., of the University of Wisconsin Medical School faculty. Dr. Samp compared the young and the old in the population sample of 7,000 to learn what he could about the road to a longer life.

"I don't have any answers, but I do have some beautiful suggestions," he laughed when we interviewed him. In Dr. Samp's research, mental attitude made a significant contribution to longevity. "The emphasis we found in older people was on a certain inner peace," he explained. "Somewhere in life, these people found living so precious. . .they wanted to live and they were willing to work at it."

Because various studies suggest that mental attitude may be a key factor in longevity, optimism is a good avenue to choose. "I think people can make themselves optimistic," said Dr. Samp. "Every morning they have the choice of getting up and saying, 'This is going to be a good day' or 'This is going to be a lousy day.' The quality of our days does not depend all that much on outside forces. The quality of our days depends on things that reside within us."

And, evidently, it's never too late to let this inside optimism out. A study of breast cancer patients in England showed that more women who had a fighting spirit after surgery remained alive and free of malignancy than women who reacted with feelings of helplessness and hopelessness (*Lancet*, October 13, 1979).

Religious People Fare Better

What's more, people who belong to a church or synagogue tend to live longer than those who do not, according to a study done in California (*American Journal of Epidemiology*, February, 1979). Other investigations have found that churchgoing Mormon men between the ages of 35 and 64 have a lower death rate than average men. That means, according to this study's figures, that at age 35 a Mormon can expect to live another 44 years, while a non-Mormon might have just 37 more (*Cancer*, October, 1978). And Seventh-day Adventists, according to still another study, have lower blood pressure and lower cholesterol levels and they weigh less (all good omens for longevity) than the general population (*Medical Journal of Australia*, May 19, 1979).

Part of the reason for the good health and long life of both the Christian groups studied may be diet. People of those particular faiths refrain from using alcohol, tobacco, coffee, tea, cola and refined foods. They are encouraged to eat fresh fruits, vegetables and whole grains, and drink milk, fruit juice and plenty of water. Seventh-day Adventists are discouraged from eating meat, and Mormons eat it in moderation. But diet and living habits are evidently only part of the explanation. Nonsmoking Adventists still develop fatal lung cancer only half as commonly as non-Adventists (*American Journal of Epidemiology*, August, 1980).

So it may be that the various social and psychological aspects of religion also contribute to health and longevity. Many social scientists agree that membership in a religious group has a beneficial effect on the nerves. For instance, Seventh-day Adventists have been found to use tranquilizers less often than other people studied, and they report fewer problems with mental illness, suicidal depressions, anxiety and tension. It could be that living within a stable network of family and friends, on top of his church affiliation, contributes toward a religious person's sense of personal worth, a quality which seems to protect health. Alienated people, it has often been shown, get sick more often and more easily than those with strong social ties.

At Madison General Hospital in Madison, Wisconsin, the Reverend Lowell Mays, Ph.D., is a psychotherapist and director of the hospital's department of human ecology. Dr. Mays told us that some people use religion to weather serious setbacks or to prevent psychosomatic illness.

"The chances of recovery from a stroke or mastectomy are much better if the person feels she is spiritually worthwhile or if she feels that life has value beyond the limitations of the body," said Dr. Mays. "If she can transcend the immediate crisis, she may have a less complicated recovery.

"Part of the Judeo-Christian tradition is taking responsibility for your own health," Dr. Mays explained further, "because you're of no use to glorify God and serve others if you aren't able and strong."

Do You Like Your Work?

Research indicates that work satisfaction is also an important aid on the road to a longer life. In 1955 a citrus farm worker named Charlie Smith had to retire because he was considered too old to be climbing trees. He was 113. But Charlie still wasn't ready to retire, so he ran a small store in Bartow, Florida, until he was 133. In 1972 he was officially recognized as the oldest person living in the United States.

At Duke University, Erdmore Palmore, Ph.D., studied a group of 270 older residents of Durham, North Carolina, and found that work satisfaction was a strong predictor of longevity, especially among men. The study defined work as jobs around the house, volunteer duties and paid employment. It was found that meaningful, satisfying work was important to longevity, because jobs offer three large benefits. First, said Dr. Palmore, jobs provide people with exercise to keep the body stimulated and functioning. Second, jobs offer mental stimulation, and third, they keep people socially active. Satisfying work gives people social support from those they respect, and praise gives people reason for respecting themselves.

Creativity Makes Long Life a Joy

Creativity and longevity also seem to go hand in hand, according to research done by Alice Dawson, Ph.D., and an associate at the United States International University in San Diego, California. In 1962, Dr. Dawson and other university psychologists compared 29 people over 65 who took up oil painting to 19 other elderly people who did not. By 1971, the oil painters had outlived their nonpainting peers almost two to one. And as might be expected, 65 percent of the painters (but only 12 percent of the nonpainters) were in good health at the end of the study. And oil painting isn't the only way to stretch life expectancy. Many of the painters were also engaged in other creative pursuits, such as photography, ceramics, needlework and teaching. The people who eschewed painting in the study also turned their backs on other creative activities (*Journal of Psychology*, vol. 82, 1972).

After all is said and done, then, emotional and spiritual health seem to count just as much as physical health in a plan for longevity. It's nice to know that we can live to a rich old age *and* enjoy getting there!

Slowing the Aging Process: The Experts Speak Out

CHAPTER **11**

Editor's Note: *To underscore our 10-point strategy for long life, we present here an encouraging report on a life-extension conference attended by Mark Bricklin, Executive Editor of Prevention magazine. Several aging and longevity researchers met in San Rafael, California, in March, 1977, to share their scientific observations—and advice for long life.*

We're driving on U.S. 101, up the Pacific Coast from Mill Valley to San Rafael, to take in a conference at the Marin Civic Center called "Slowing the Aging Process: Life Extension and the Control of Aging."

It's early in the morning and as we begin rolling north, the scenery is dominated by a great brawny creature called Mount Tamalpais, shrouded in ragged, gunmetal gray clouds. They tell me Mt. Tamalpais is sacred to the Indians, a *healing* mountain. A few moments later the sun begins to break through and the long green base of the mountain is dappled with incredibly bright sunlight. A good omen, I tell myself.

I'm shocked when we reach the Marin Auditorium and Civic Center. They're actually beautiful, probably the first such large public buildings I've ever seen that project really pleasant feelings. Behind them rise mountains. Palm trees and duck ponds in front. Inside, it's even better. The rows of seats—can you believe it?—are actually far enough apart so that you can stretch your legs! Looking forward to two solid days' worth of sitting at this conference, that extra leg room seems to me a stroke of genius. A staff member of the Wholistic Health Nutrition Institute of Mill Valley, which is presenting the conference, tells me that the buildings were designed by Frank Lloyd Wright. Ah, my favorite architect: the practical visionary who called his work "organic architecture." He wanted it to be an integral part of nature instead of something rudely, synthetically imposed on the scene. The same philosophy we follow at Rodale Press, with our organic gardening and organic lifestyle.

During the next two days as I relax in my organic chair, it seems that most of the speakers take a kind of organic approach to the practical side of life extension. In fact, many of them, after summing up their years of research, recommend steps that are remarkably similar to what *Prevention* magazine recommends.

For sure, all these experts are well aware of the extremely artificial experimental approaches to longevity which are being studied today, such as putting laboratory rats on unnatural and severely restrictive diets from the moment they are weaned, and even taking aim at the chemical makeup of our very chromosomes in hopes that we can fool them into thinking we are 18 when we're really 58. But right now, and maybe for a long time to come, using such approaches on human beings would only succeed in getting the experimenter thrown into jail.

But there is much to be gained—many years of vigorous, healthful life—by following the commonsense advice offered by some of today's experts on longevity.

You Can Choose to Live Longer

Many people probably think that how long you live (barring accidents) is determined by your heredity—your chromosomes. But the truth seems to be that while you may indeed enjoy about the same number of years of life as your parents, the reason for that isn't only a result of the genetic material they passed along to you, but their *way of living*.

That was brought home clearly by Hardin B. Jones, Ph.D., one of the pioneers and leading authorities in the field of aging, and professor of medical physics and physiology at the University of California at Berkeley.

Consider, Dr. Jones suggested, a man who gets no exercise, is overweight, smokes, drinks, is single, and lives in New York City. Contrast him with a man who is active, slender, doesn't drink, is married, lives in a rural area and is a citizen of one of the Scandinavian countries. What would you guess to be the difference in their average life expectancy? Five years? Ten years? As much, perhaps, as 20? Actually, the difference in their life expectancy is fully 37 years!

What's happening here is not that the Scandinavian has somehow extended the upper limit of longevity. Rather, the New Yorker, with all his bad health and social habits, who lives in a crowded and polluted city, has done just about everything possible to *shorten* his life expectancy. And just as important, he has reduced the *quality* of his life. As Dr. Jones puts it, "A typical Swedish man at 90 is physiologically like we are at 60."

To take a closer look at the subject of aging, Dr. Jones pointed out that in infancy all parts of our body are nourished by about the same flow of blood. But as we grow older, our circulation slows down, and most of the nourishment is directed toward our organs, while our muscles and connective tissues get less and less.

To illustrate the extent of this change, Dr. Jones said that at the age of 12, each liter (about a quart) of our muscle tissue receives 50 milliliters of blood per minute while resting. By 18, that figure has dropped to 25 milliliters, and by the age of 30, all the way down to 10!

That sounds a little grim, but the good news is that in athletes this change simply does not take place. Moral: Exercise is the single best thing you can do to keep young. It not only helps prevent most major arterial diseases, but gives the heart that *reserve* of strength it needs to get us past a crisis.

If exercise is the best thing you can do, the *worst* thing you can do is to smoke. Smoking not only cripples the circulatory system, but is responsible, in Dr. Jones's estimation, for fully 70 percent of all cancers in our society. And if you want to compound the damage of smoking, let yourself become fat and drink a lot. (For what they'll do to you, see Dr. Jones's book, *Sensual Drugs*, Cambridge University Press, 1977.)

It's curious, Dr. Jones suggested, that people are very concerned about such signs of aging as white hair and wrinkles—which do not limit our life in the least—while they often ignore basic health habits which in the end will make or break us.

Optimize Health with Supplements

And, Professor Jones declared in answer to a question from the audience, "I am sure in favor of taking vitamin supplements."

That advice was echoed by several other experts on life extension, including Chadd Everone, Ph.D., who's affiliated with a number of major universities and is a governing trustee of the

Foundation of Infinite Survival, an unusual organization which studies the theoretical and practical aspects of life extension.

Ideally, Dr. Everone suggested, we all ought to get "advance data" on such fundamental things as our blood flow, the condition of our arteries and blood vessels, our hearing, glucose tolerance, and dietary pattern. Within five or ten years, he predicted, we will be able to look at our genes and understand what their structure tells us, so that we can see if we have a predisposition to develop certain problems. Taking all this information into account, we would then aggressively embark on a series of programs to stop or even reverse any deterioration.

But there are a number of good things we can do right now, he emphasized. First on his list was to take nutritional supplements, as they will "optimize your health." He also suggested cutting down on fat and sugar, as well as avoiding food additives. Cigarettes and liquor should also be avoided.

Get plenty of exercise, he urged, the kind that makes you breathe hard but feel good. Avoid undue stress. Avoid unneeded radiation, from x-rays. To help control your intake of toxins, Dr. Everone suggests drinking filtered or distilled water. If you drink distilled water, he added, use mineral supplements to restore the vital nutrients distilling removes along with toxins.

I ought to add here that not all the speakers were in favor of taking vitamins. One, a very distinguished scientist whom I will not mention by name, said he was very skeptical about the idea that vitamin E could slow the aging process. I think that was his polite way of saying that he thought all vitamins were just a lot of rubbish. Curiously, the same speaker announced that he had eaten a candy bar first thing in the morning to give him quick energy (the audience groaned). He also defended saccharin, urging the audience to keep using it. And as far as I was able to tell, he was the only speaker who, off the platform, smoked cigarettes—rather heavily at that.

Hans Kugler, Ph.D., on the other hand, is a robust young biochemist who believes that smoking cigarettes is "sucking on death." He is also another firm believer in vitamin supplementation, to achieve longer life. Or more accurately, to extend whatever potential we have for longevity and its natural upper limits.

Eating Better, Living Longer

Dr. Kugler, a consultant on aging who lives in Los Angeles, explained that he has demonstrated with laboratory animals the truth of what many of the speakers said about the importance of health habits. Using mice which had already reached maturity, he put them on one of a number of programs devised to reflect various lifestyles and dietary patterns. One group of animals, for instance, which he dubbed "Average Businessmen," were fed a diet similar to that eaten by many human beings (containing 20 percent refined sugar), were not exercised, received the alcohol equivalent of four strong drinks a day, and were subjected to cigarette smoke once a day for about an hour.

At the other end of the scale was a group of animals who were exercised in a rotating drum twice a week, given a more interesting environment, and supplemented with brewer's yeast, wheat germ, dolomite, vitamin C and B complex. They were also given a large amount of vitamin E.

The last group, Kugler told me, lived an average of more than 50 percent longer (after the programs were begun) than the first group.

Recently, Dr. Kugler has been analyzing dietary and lifestyle surveys which are scored with the help of a computer, and he has found that remarkably few people are doing everything they can to optimize their life span. He's also found some interesting correlations between diet and behavior. For instance, he reported, the dietary survey revealed that 90 percent of the respondents who said they were taking tranquilizers had a low intake of magnesium—a mineral known to be important to the health of the nervous system.

Mice, Horses—Why Not People?

Although it's hard—even for an enthusiastic scientist like Dr. Kugler—to optimize a human being's lifestyle the way you can that of a laboratory mouse, he did put some of his theories into action with a *horse.*

"We went to this stable to buy a riding horse and were looking at a very handsome animal, when someone jokingly suggested that we buy a horse that was obviously in terrible health. Its rear legs were so swollen from kicking that they looked like telephone poles. The asking price was only $200—a fraction of what most of the other horses cost—and, on an impulse, we bought it."

Over a period of months, he went on, he gave the horse plenty of loving attention, plenty of vitamins, and all the other good things that people ought to get. The result was that this "joke" of a horse won six ribbons in one day competing against horses that had sold for 10 to 20 times as much.

It's worth keeping in mind that this horse received plenty of love along with his vitamins. And, in fact, most of the same speakers at this conference who recommended vitamins also emphasized the importance of love, affection and good relationships with others.

One of those was Peter Keagan, a brilliant and internationally recognized innovator in the design of homes, villages and cities. Affiliated with the Energy Conservation Institute, Keagan detailed some of the components of what he considered to be a healthier lifestyle for people and the entire ecosystem.

Vitamin therapy and exposure to full-spectrum sunlight were two of the specific things he thought were good for people. He then went on to detail why it's important for us to use alternative supplies of energy, and explained how we should make greater use of waterpower, solar energy, geothermal energy and other technologies and energies that do not pollute the earth and exhaust natural resources.

"But," he cautioned, "we must never lose sight of the fact that with all these systems, people do matter. . . .

"Love is the key energy. All other energies are secondary."

Index